If You Can't/Won't Stop Smoking

If You Can't / Won't Stop Smoking

How to Reduce the Ill Effects of Tobacco

Dr. James Scala

St. Martin's Press New York

DESIGN BY DIANE STEVENSON / SNAP•HAUS GRAPHICS

Library of Congress Cataloging-in-Publication Data

Scala, James, 1934–
    If you can't/won't stop smoking : how to reduce the ill effects
of tobacco / James Scala.
        p.   cm.
    ISBN 0-312-08141-3
    1. Smoking—Health aspects.   I. Title.
RA1242.T6S23   1993
616.86'5—dc20   92-26282
                                                            CIP

First Edition: January 1993

10 9 8 7 6 5 4 3 2 1

To Louise:
No man could hope for a better sister than you.
Since you can't stop smoking,
please follow the teachings in this book.
James Scala

CONTENTS

ACKNOWLEDGMENTS

Al Zuckerman: We seldom meet a man who can make a commitment and not look back. Al is that man.

Kimberly Scala, my daughter: Thanks for doing the tedious task of compiling and organizing the references. You did a great job!

Nancy Scala, my wife: You keep proving that you can accomplish anything as long as you don't care who gets the credit.

Maureen Baron and Michelle Levy: Thanks for getting behind this project and letting me do my job. You will have helped many people.

PREFACE

would like all smokers and tobacco users to quit, but I'd also like all overweight people to slim down and those with high blood pressure to diet and exercise correctly so their blood pressure can become normal. Everyone also should stop using alcoholic beverages to excess. While I'm at it, I should call a stop to unsafe sex, drug use, dishonest politicians, and so on. But life's not like that, and I'm not sure humanity would move ahead if it was.

Some people can stop smoking, and I hope they will. Others will never stop smoking. Even though the primary audience for this book is those who *won't* stop smoking, people who do stop can still benefit from its teachings because the effects of smoking linger.

Still others can benefit from this book. People who love smokers think that living with them is worth the extra health risk of breathing passive smoke. And children living in a smoking household have no choice. This book is also for anyone who lives, works, or plays with a smoker.

Chewing tobacco has become widespread in recent years. Young people who chew tobacco usually stop by about age thirty-five. Others, however, won't ever stop. This book can help both groups because, as with smoking, the effects of tobacco linger even after people quit chewing.

The advice in this book also can help a wider range of Americans—anyone who is forced to breathe less-than-pure air. People who live and work in cities or work around smoke, solvents, and chemicals have similar health problems to those of smokers. These people, too, can benefit by following the recommendations in this book. They will gain a longer, healthier life.

WHY SMOKE?

The idea for this book actually grew out of a comment I heard on the radio. I was listening to Dr. Dean Edell answer medical questions, and he asked: "Have you ever wondered why people smoke? In the face of adverse publicity, they keep it up.

Does smoking have something going for it?" I went to the library that day with those questions on my mind.

When I read that 1,631,540 cigarettes are lit up every minute, I too asked: "Why?" I learned that smoking has some positive effects for many people. In fact, I was so fascinated by its positive effects that I wrote Chapter 16 to help folks understand themselves and people who smoke. These positive effects are pronounced in some people. We all know someone who is easier to get along with if he or she smokes. More research into these positive effects is needed.

I came home from the library that day recognizing that many people will always smoke. Thus it follows that many people will live and work with smokers. Also, because many people must live and work in places where the air isn't pure, they encounter the same ill health effects as smokers. I challenged myself that day and asked: "How can I help people minimize the effects of smoking, tobacco use, and bad air?" This book is the result.

NOT FOR WOMEN ONLY

Two chapters deal specifically with women's issues: Chapter 9, on osteoporosis, a disease that affects women almost exclusively, and Chapter 10, on pregnancy.

The best way to deal with osteoporosis, or thinning of the bones, is through prevention. Women are naturally prone to osteoporosis, and smoking increases a women's chances of coming down with the disease. Osteoporosis means "porous bones." It's a disease in which calcium is slowly lost from the bones, causing them to become porous, thin, and to shatter easily. Diet and food supplements, however, can reduce the risks imposed by smoking. When a little exercise is added, there's a good chance that the risk of osteoporosis can be completely eliminated.

However, when you smoke, pregnancy is a special situation. Although I promised myself that I wouldn't preach in this book, I strongly suggest that every woman make a special effort to quit or, at the least, reduce smoking and any other tobacco use during the period before conception and during pregnancy. (Note that it is important to quit even *before* you become pregnant.) Yet I know that many women will not stop or even cut back on smoking during pregnancy. Chapter 10 provides good advice for any would-be mother who smokes or lives with a smoker.

BEAUTY ISN'T SKIN DEEP

Because smoking has a definite influence on the color, tone, and wrinkles of skin, it most certainly affects a smoker's looks. Tone refers to the "leathery" feel of skin that people talk about regarding smokers. These effects are real, scientists have studied them, and we have a pretty good understanding of what causes them. Consequently, we can explain how smokers can slow down these skin problems. Even if you follow the steps in this book out of vanity alone, just to gain better skin color and hair sheen, every organ in your body will benefit. I'll have succeeded, and you'll be a winner.

CHEWING TOBACCO

Although the main focus is on smoking, my words also apply to tobacco chewers, with a couple of exceptions. Chewers, or "snuff dippers," avoid a few risks, but take on other equally serious risks.

Dippers avoid lung cancer because they don't smoke. But they are at high risk for the various forms of mouth cancer, including tongue, esophagus, cheek, and gum cancer. In fact, I suspect that dippers are at a higher risk of getting mouth cancer compared to average folk than smokers are at risk of getting lung cancer compared to nonsmokers.

Additionally, snuff dippers have a higher risk of digestive-system cancer. Although the statistics aren't available, the preliminary data suggests tobacco chewers have the same risks as smokers, with the possible exception of some causes of heart disease. Snuff dippers have a lower risk of heart disease than smokers because they avoid the oxidative damage that starts heart disease. However, their risks of high blood pressure and high cholesterol are the same or greater than those of smokers.

So, with those few exceptions, this book applies to snuff dippers as well as to smokers. If they follow the diet plans, supplement recommendations, and exercise programs, they will benefit as much as smokers.

FOR CHILDREN

Children have no choice—if a parent smokes, they smoke. If a mother smokes during pregnancy, the baby smokes. Similarly, children who live in cities effectively smoke. So the plans and advice in this book are for them as well. Just apply some common sense regarding dosage and portion size.

If adults need extra antioxidant nutrients and vegetables, so do children. They should use the supplements in proportion to their size. Food-serving size will take care of the rest. Children will benefit from my teachings more than their parents and will have a better chance at a healthy, disease-free life. Isn't that the best way to try to make things better for our children?

IF YOU CAN'T/WON'T STOP SMOKING

REDUCING RISKS

I n his log of 1492, Columbus wrote about many Indian practices. Of one he said: "They packed a tube called a tabac with an herb, lit one end, and drank smoke from the other end." Columbus saw no practical value to "drinking" smoke and said no more. In contrast, he also noticed the hammock, which he brought back to Spain as a practical invention. In dismissing the smoking habit, he misjudged a human tendency to enjoy tobacco that became an enormous, worldwide industry.

Dr. Ronald Siegel, a world-known expert on human addiction, claims tobacco use is over eight thousand years old. Over the centuries, reactions toward it have varied. Tobacco was outlawed at times and encouraged at other times. In the early twentieth century, smoking was widely accepted. Until the late 1950s, in fact, some physicians considered it good for you and even recommended it to "melancholic" patients. Veteran Administration doctors occasionally prescribed menthol cigarettes for combined cases of lethargy and nasal congestion.

Because smoking was viewed as a pleasure, tobacco has been taxed in most countries since about the sixteenth century. By the 1980s, when scientists agreed that smoking was bad for your health, it was looked upon as a vice and the effort to force people to quit smoking created a reason for more taxes. Now that people who don't smoke have decided that smoking is offensive, a third tax base has developed.

You can't fight taxes, but you can fight the risks tobacco imposes on your health by making modest changes in your eating, food supplement, and exercise habits. If routinely practiced, these changes will help you feel better, look better, and live longer, because your risk of tobacco-related illnesses will decline. Making these changes also will help some people reduce their guilt load.

ANOTHER VIEW

Because the health risks associated with smoking receive so much publicity, everyone simply tells smokers to quit. No one seems to ask: Could there be a compromise? Is there something the smoker can do to reduce risk and still smoke? The answers to those two questions might surprise some people. Smoking does indeed carry risks, but these risks are interrelated, and they can be reduced by eating the correct food and making some life-style changes.

Lung cancer, the most publicized risk, is a case in point. Japanese smokers have about half the lung cancer rate of American smokers in spite of the fact that the Japanese smoke more cigarettes that are stronger and have more tar. Based on these facts, you would expect the Japanese lung cancer rate to be higher than ours in North America. Their reduced rate of lung cancer defies the concept of one habit (smoking) = one risk (lung cancer).

Dietary differences explain the lower lung cancer rate in Japan. The Japanese diet is rich in antioxidant foods, and green tea and black tea, widely used as beverages, have a special, preventive effect. Americans drink comparable amounts of coffee, which has no health benefits. Animal studies on diet and specific nutrients in which the Japanese diet is rich support these concepts. Thus these lab studies support the anecdotal evidence, even though solid, replicable experiments may be lacking at this time.

Original smoking studies in the United States and England showed that risk of cancer was in proportion to the amount of cigarettes smoked and their tar content. These studies also showed that the rates of lung cancer among some people who smoked was just a little higher than for those folks who didn't smoke. Why?

The answer is simple. Those smokers who didn't get cancer, on average, ate foods rich in protective substances called antioxidants. Antioxidants dramatically reduce the risk of cancer, heart disease, and other less spectacular illnesses, such as cataracts. In addition these people's diets included three other protector substances: the B vitamins, vitamin E, vitamin C. Besides protecting them from lung cancer, these same substances and food habits reduced other risks that smoking exaggerates.

RISK IS PART OF LIVING

Tobacco use has risks as do most things we do. Most smokers are aware of smoking's health risks; they accept them without giving them much thought. In contrast, many things we do regularly have risks that most of us don't recognize, and if we do, we accept them. We add risks to our life when we eat some staple foods—such as meats (fat) and fish (potential toxins)—that are the very foundation of our diet. Some risk always accompanies medication use, even from drugs prescribed to restore health or keep us alive. We increase our risk of arthritis when we exercise, even though our intention is to keep trim and prevent heart disease. In life we trade one risk for another and think it's a good deal, if we think about it at all.

When you take an aspirin, for example, who tells you to take some vitamin C and fish oils to counter its negative side effects? We're repeatedly told to reduce fat; the national American average of about 40 percent of calories from fat is far above the recommended 30 percent or less calories from fat. School lunch programs often contain high-fat foods, such as hot dogs and sausage pizza, yet who tells parents to serve kids a vegetarian meal later on? When we barbecue or smoke fish or meat, do we consider that the cooking processes create some carcinogens? No, because we like the flavor this type of cooking imparts to the food.

Just as many people are willing to accept the risks offered

by aspirins, high-fat foods, and even barbecued and smoked meats, smoking carries some risks that many people are willing to accept. The problem is, in comparison, tobacco use carries a larger, more well-defined spectrum of risks than most of these other habits. Indeed, smoking risks are so well defined and unique that life insurance companies charge smokers higher rates than nonsmokers. (At age forty, male smokers pay 32 percent more and female smokers, 20 percent more, than nonsmokers. Smoking is a single, identifiable, well-documented habit. Heredity, overweight, drinking, and other activities are often more deadly, but they are more difficult to define and easier to hide from the insurance companies.

Let's examine why smoking risks seem so clear and see what positive steps you can take to reduce them if you decide to keep smoking.

HOW HEALTH RISKS ARE DECIDED

Epidemiologists are medical detectives who work with large numbers of people and powerful computers. These detectives asked a basic question: What causes lung cancer? They then identified the life-style habits of thousands of people with lung cancer and paired each person with someone of the same age, living in the same area, who didn't have lung cancer. They got as close a match as possible and minimized basic demographic differences to focus on life-style habits. From matching millions of such pairs, they identified one habit that predisposed toward lung cancer: smoking. The fact that the epidemiologists found other activities that reduced the risk of smoking went largely unnoticed outside academic circles.

Think about how many individual differences there are between people and you can see why these scientists needed myriad pairs and powerful computers. For example, besides the obvious ethnic-genetic differences, such minor differences as exercise, amount of smoking, drinking, the consumption of vegetables, fruit, meat, and fish, and so on, also exist. To carry this further, add minor variations. For example, vegetables are separated into green, yellow, white, cruciferous, bulbs, and so on. Consequently, there's a lot of information to sort through, and it changes as trends start to appear.

From these extensive evaluations, the scientist found a number of factors that predispose toward lung cancer. We call these factors risks. Risks can be negative or positive. You already know that smoking increases lung cancer risk, but so does living in a city, driving regularly in heavy traffic, or working with chemicals, such as asbestos and solvents. One habit that reduces lung cancer risk involves eating vegetables rich in antioxidants.

The risk factor associated with smoking varies depending on the number of cigarettes smoked, types of tobacco, filters, types of filters, and so on. Chewing tobacco also is a serious risk with variations, such as amount chewed, method of chewing, additives in the tobacco, and so on. Thus even a clear-cut risk is not as well defined as we're often led to believe. Similarly it is not clear and simple how much of a risk reducer, such as eating vegetables, is needed to produce a protective effect.

Once the epidemiologists discovered that smoking increased cancer risk and vegetables decreased it, myriad new questions emerged about risk reduction. Which vegetables? Are more vegetables better, or is it selected vegetables? What about fruit? Is there a relationship between the number of cigarettes and the servings of vegetables? There's simply no end to the questions. Nailing down the details could keep many research scientists busy for decades.

Unfortunately, when smoking surfaced as a positive risk for lung cancer, scientists and policymakers took a direct, easy approach and said, "quit smoking." As the taxes on it prove, smoking has always been considered something you didn't *need* to do. By taking this one-sided approach, policymakers didn't bother to spell out the other side of the story: that by following a good diet, taking the correct supplements, and exercising, the risk of lung cancer can be reduced.

WHAT EPIDEMIOLOGISTS HAVE LEARNED

Sure, epidemiologists have confirmed what we already know: Smoking, living with a smoker, or working in a city with poor air increases many health risks. However, many of these health risks also increase with age and a poor diet. For example, if you could live in an idyllic Garden of Eden, you'd still have a risk of developing cancer, heart disease, or cataracts, to name just a few, as you got older. "It's life," as they say. But smoking accelerates all of these risks and makes them worse.

Tobacco use increases the risk of most cancer and accelerates many illnesses often called "diseases of aging." By correcting your life-style habits, you can reduce the rate at which these risks accumulate. Some susceptibilities, such as the risk of cataracts, even can be reduced to less than that of nonsmokers. Table 1.1 summarizes the most pertinent risks.

TABLE 1.1
TOBACCO USE RISKS THAT CAN BE REDUCED BY DIET AND LIFE-STYLE CHANGES

Cosmetic	Cancer	Diseases of Aging
Age spots	Aerodigestive	Asthma
Eye clarity	(mouth, esophagus, etc.)	Cataracts
Gum tone	Bladder	Emphysema
Hair sheen	Colonic	Heart disease
Poor fingernails	Leukemia	Hypertension
Skin color	Lung	Nasal polyps
Skin wrinkles	Pancreatic	Osteoporosis
	Rectal	Periodontal disease
		Ulcers

Table 1.1 is the bare bones; it doesn't tell the whole story. Most risks result from the oxidative toxins in smoke, which cause cellular damage and many other risks are secondary to them. Table 1.2 shows the problems that can be reduced by selecting foods rich in antioxidants and taking food supplements.

TABLE 1.2
RISKS RELATED TO INSUFFICIENT ANTIOXIDANTS

Cosmetic	Cancer	Aging
Age spots	Aerodigestive	Cataracts
Skin color	Bladder	Emphysema
Skin wrinkles	Colon and rectal	Heart Disease
	Lung	Hypertension
	Pancreatic	

The risks emphasized in Table 1.1 are derived from a combination of the metabolic effects of smoking and the oxidating and irritating effects of smoking. These also can be reduced by eating the correct food, taking food supplements, and exercising. By doing so, your life-style will give you a good chance at normal health. Consider this example: Because you smoke, your risk of bladder cancer is above the national average. Lycopene, a carotenoid in tomatoes, red fruits, and vegetables, reduces the risk of bladder cancer. Eating foods rich in lycopene regularly reduces your risk of bladder cancer to near average, so a daily serving of pasta with tomato sauce, a salad with tomatoes or red peppers, a slice of watermelon, or snacking on picante sauce is an easy preventive step to take. Thus the foods you eat can reduce your risk of cancer.

SMOKERS DON'T USUALLY EAT A GOOD DIET

Epidemiologists learn many things about people, including smokers, and the information can be viewed from many vantage points. Each vantage point helps build a creative strategy to offset smoking's health risks. So, consider the typical smoker's dietary shortfalls.

Since only 9 percent of people eat the required five servings of fruits and vegetables daily, you can see that smokers aren't alone in not following a balanced and varied diet. It's just that they are a little worse than the average, and their smoking habit dictates that they should be better than average.

Research published in such prestigious medical journals as the *American Journal of Clinical Nutrition* and the *American Journal of Public Health*, among others, have reported the following:

- Smokers eat too much meat.
- Smokers don't eat as many fruits and vegetables as nonsmokers.
- Smokers don't eat as much cereal as nonsmokers.
- Smokers eat far too few cruciferous vegetables.
- Smokers are likely to consume more coffee and alcohol than nonsmokers.
- Smokers are likely to be short in vitamins A, C, E, folic acid, several other B vitamins, and the minerals calcium, selenium, and zinc.

Smokers need more nutrients, especially antioxidants and antixiodant nutrients, such as vitamins E and C, than average folks, and diet surveys prove they are getting less. As a group, smokers need more protective cruciferous vegetables, such as broccoli and cabbage, and they eat less. They definitely need more fiber than average folks, and they get less. This evidence suggests they should choose tea, limit coffee, and drink more fruit and vegetable juices. Their snacks should be such things as carrots, fruit, and dishes with picante sauce.

I already told you about Japanese smokers, and how they have a lower incidence of lung cancer than Americans. But they also have a lower risk for everything else on Table 1.1. When all differences between American and Japanese smokers are considered, it comes down to diet, because other Japanese life-style habits, such as exercise, are even worse than ours. Their low-fat, more vegetarianlike diet is better than ours by a long stretch.

In the United States, smokers' diets contribute significantly to their risk. Look back to Table 1.1. Certain illnesses, such as various cancers, cataracts, and hypertension, are more related to diet than to smoking. And we do know from studying smokers ad nauseam that they don't select their food correctly.

If all that's not enough, only 23.1 percent of American adults use a daily food supplement whether they smoke or not. All smokers need supplements regularly, and occasional use isn't good enough. Smokers need above-average levels of all nutrients and significantly more of the B vitamins and the antioxidant nutrients, which include vitamins C, E, and beta carotene. They also can get additional protective benefits from other selected vegetables, additional fiber, and fish that are rich in the right oils.

These nutritional shortfalls, as I call them, aren't great enough for you to notice them or for your doctor to diagnose them as a deficiency. However, these shortfalls accumulate over the years. For instance, this is one reason why women who smoke are more likely to develop osteoporosis. It also explains why smoking accelerates the onset of cataracts and why bladder cancer is more likely among smokers. Eating correctly costs no more and can pay excellent dividends for everyone, especially smokers.

WHEN TO START ON YOUR ANTIRISK DIET

Start now! Whenever I speak to a group of people who smoke or use tobacco, I'm asked something like this: "Dr. Scala, I've been smoking for over twenty years, so what's the point of starting a new health program now?" My answer is always the same: "Time after time, research has conclusively proven that your body can improve at any age. Since this is the first instant of the rest of your life, now is the best time to start. It doesn't matter if you're nineteen or ninety years of age. Start now!"

GETTING AN EARLY START

I've already mentioned a few ways to reduce risks and explained that, as a smoker, you are likely to eat less fruits and vegetables than nonsmokers, even though you need more. I also said smokers need more nutrients. Remember the following simple rules the next time you snack or prepare a meal.

- Drink two glasses of orange juice or eat two oranges, two cups of strawberries, or two kiwi fruit every day.
- Eat some red fruits or vegetables every day; for example, a tomato salad, tomato sauce, red pepper, watermelon, or all of them.
- Have seven servings of fruits and vegetables daily. Fruit is usually expressed as a single piece, such as an apple, pear, or peach; if it's served cut up, it should be at least a half cup. Vegetables are usually served in half-cup portions, although the serving could be a large broccoli spear or about six, small asparagus spears.
- Make sure at least one serving of vegetables or fruit is orange or yellow. Eat carrots, yellow or red beans, sweet potatoes, a slice of cantaloupe, or papaya.
- Snack at least once daily on a raw carrot and don't count it as either a fruit or vegetable; think of it as insurance. If you like a dip, go for picante sauce or salsa.
- Supplements: Take a multivitamin-multimineral supplement each day and be sure it provides 100 percent of the Recommended Dietary Allowance (RDA) for all nutrients, except calcium and magnesium. It should contain at least 10 percent of the RDA for calcium and magnesium as well. Then take enough specific calcium-magnesium supplements to get 100 percent of the RDA for each. A few good products are listed in Chapter 17.

CHAPTER TWO

BLOCKING TOXINS FROM SMOKE

L ife depends on oxygen in the air. We see oxygen's ability to fuel oxidation whenever we strike a match, start our car, launch a rocket, or see a rusty nail. We use the same process with every breath we take. In contrast to these flaming examples, however, oxidative processes in our body take place at body temperature and faster than the rocket launch or auto engine startup. If our body worked at the snail's pace of rust, we'd be long gone.

The by-products of the oxidation process are the same in all these cases: carbon dioxide and water. You can see the water drip from your car's exhaust or surround the rocket's blast. All of these processes are fueled by very similar chemicals, whether it's an auto engine or human food. Fats are chemically very much like gasoline, and carbohydrates, because they are partly oxidized in the plant that makes them, differ only slightly. The most important question is: How does the same process occur at body temperature that goes on at hundreds of degrees in engines? Or, how does it occur so fast in our body compared to the slow oxidation rate of rust?

The instant you breathe in, your blood traps oxygen with iron (like the rusty nail) and transports it to all body tissues, where it's passed on to your body's 50 trillion cells. In these cells, the oxygen combines with carbon and hydrogen. The carbon combines with oxygen to make carbon dioxide; hydrogen is passed to oxygen to make water; and both chemical actions release energy (burning), just as they do in the rocket blast. The instant you breathe out, you release the wastes (carbon dioxide and water). You can't see the carbon dioxide, but on a cold day you can see the water, as vapor, when you exhale.

Our body performs this miracle through the elaborate process we call metabolism. Metabolism is made to happen by enzymes, natural catalysts that lower the energy barriers, like the spark plug in a car or the friction to strike a match. Many enzymes work to make oxidation occur at body temperature, not at the hundreds of degrees required by man-made processes. The remarkable human body is able to extract more energy from a pound of fuel than even the most advanced man-made engines. Not only does nature perform the same processes at body temperature, but it's more efficient as well.

Don't be surprised that your body is more efficient than an auto engine. Your body represents just over four billion years that life has been developing on earth, and most forms of life have been using oxygen for over two billion of those years. That's a lot of time for nature to test many options and decide which ones work well. Because evolution continues, you can bet that life will become even more efficient as time goes on.

But what about the rusty nail? Rust is a natural process, yet it is unwanted and illustrates that some forms of oxidation are bad.

OXIDATION ISN'T ALWAYS GOOD

While oxidation is essential to life and the convenience of getting around by car, it's not always wanted. For instance, we don't want the car or the nail to rust out. Other common types of oxidations that we try to prevent are cooking oils going rancid, opened wine spoiling, an apple turning brown, and so on.

The simplest way to prevent oxidation is to shut out oxygen. For example, we cover a jar of oil so the air can't get to it, paint the fender on a car, or galvanize a nail. We also can slow the oxidation process down by refrigerating oils and even freezing foods. Alternatively, we can introduce a

material that reacts with the oxygen more easily. By sacrific-
ing something to react with the oxygen, we are "trapping"
oxygen in something else.

Let's consider an apple. Slice an apple in half and set
half on the counter. Squeeze some lemon juice onto the other
half and put it alongside the first half. Antioxidants in the
lemon juice will react with oxygen in the air and keep it from
attacking the apple until they all are used up. In contrast,
the apple half without the lemon juice turns brown more
quickly because there are no antioxidants covering it. Any of
these materials that react more easily with oxygen than the
apple substances are called antioxidants.

In our environment, many things can cause unwanted
oxidation. All living things must resist these oxidizing agents
to survive. Indeed, our body depends on an elaborate system
of antioxidants to protect itself, just as we protect metal,
cooking oil, and food. Natural barriers, such as skin, saliva,
and tears, form a primary defense to keep these oxidative
materials out of our body. However, many oxidants get by the
barriers, so nature's main, secondary strategy is to sacrifice
other materials—internal antioxidants—to neutralize oxidative reactions.

ANTIOXIDANTS: NATURE'S DEMOLITION EXPERTS

Oxidants cause unwanted oxidation. Oxygen is the main oxidant, but there are many others, such as nitrates, carbon
monoxide, chlorinated hydrocarbons, superoxides, and so
on. Because an intermediate step in the oxidizing process
that involves free radicals occurs, unwanted oxidation in the
body can be neutralized. By attacking oxidation at this intermediate stage, living systems can gain the upper hand and
thrive.

In any oxidation process, atoms are shifted from one
material to another. This is done by shifting their electrons
in much the same way electrons flow in the wires of your
home to make lamps light. When desirable electron transfers
take place, the process is carefully controlled and the atoms
are not released until the process is complete. This is because

there's an intermediate stage when the oxidizing agent, usually oxygen, has an electron that isn't attached correctly. This atom with the extra electron is known as a radical. In summary, oxidative processes in the body use oxygen radicals as an important step in energy production.

When unwanted oxidation occurs, a similar radical is produced, but it's not well ordered and tightly held within the matrix of the living cell. Indeed, you can think of it as "loose" and looking for attachment at any cost. This loose, or free, radical is not planned and organized in the biological system. If the free radical combines with an important material, it can do irreparable, even deadly, damage. We say a free radical is highly reactive because nature must combine the atom with something very quickly to maintain harmony.

Free radicals—these intermediate stages of oxidation—are so reactive that scientists speak about their lifetimes in nanoseconds, or millionths of a second. Free radicals react more quickly than the best explosive, even though they are the size of atoms. Think of free radicals as superexplosives that can destroy small, essential parts of a living system. These reactions take place at the molecular level, so we can't even watch them with the most powerful microscope. All we can do is assess the accumulated damage of myriad reactions later on when they show up as a health defect, such as heart disease, cancer, cataracts, or emphysema.

Free radicals react most easily with fatty chemicals that form the membranes of cells. These fatty materials often have "unsaturated" regions that are full of electrons. Because the free radical is usually short one electron, it reacts with these materials that have an abundance of electrons. Once this reaction occurs, new unwanted chemicals are produced and the normally well-organized cell membrane has a flaw. This "flaw" is a break in nature's first defense line.

Other natural processes, such as radiation, produce free radicals directly. For example, visible light produces some free radicals that are essential for photosynthesis, the basis of all food. But ultraviolet light (UV) produces unwanted free radicals, so plants must have antioxidants whose major role is to neutralize them. Nature has made a wise choice in this strategy of neutralizing free radicals, because just about every unwanted oxidative reaction, must pass through this intermediate stage.

Further, all free radicals need to neutralize their electrons. They are different only in location of their electrons. So, by placing free-radical neutralizers—the antioxidants—in vulnerable locations, one natural strategy can stop all unwanted oxidative processes. The strategy simply calls for many antioxidants, which are plentiful in nature.

Over the years scientists have called antioxidants by many different names. "Free-radical scavengers" and "natural reducing agents" were popular at one time. "Antioxidant" has caught on recently and is used widely.

Green plants have always needed antioxidants to prevent the free radicals from ultraviolet light from causing damage. Some of these antioxidants, such as beta carotene, are essential to protect the process of photosynthesis; others, such as ascorbic acid (vitamin C), protect fruit from damage, and vitamin E protects the oils in nuts and seeds. Because humans came along after plants, we depend on many antioxidants found in plants and especially the foods we derive from them. Indeed, some foods, such as carrots, cabbage, and pumpkins, probably owe their widespread cultivation to their supply of antioxidants.

WHAT CAN FREE RADICALS DO?

Free radicals react with biochemicals that are essential to life processes. These essential biochemicals can be materials circulating in our blood, holding tissues together, components of a living cell, even the very genetic material that allows a cell to reproduce and build new tissue or produce a child. Damage done by oxidizing agents is both important and insidious. Let's take what's "important" first and consider what's "insidious" later.

When a free radical interacts with something in our blood or any body fluid, it can produce a foreign material that may be toxic, a toxin. If a cancer-causing toxin is produced, we might expect big trouble later on; or if it's a rancid oil in place of one we need, it could gum up a natural metabolic process, sort of the way a broken-down car causes bridge traffic to back up even on routes other than those leading directly to the bridge.

Once a toxin is produced our body must get rid of it, or we can expect trouble. Getting rid of the toxin means passing it through our excretory system, including our kidneys, bladder, and the intestinal tract. If we continue producing the toxin we increase the chances of overwhelming our other defenses, and our risk from the toxin's effects—for example, the chances it can cause cancer or high blood pressure—will increase. So the longer we expose ourselves to the oxidizing agent without neutralizing it or the toxins it can produce, the greater our risk.

Another frequent site of attack might be an essential component of the delicate cell membrane. If this membrane is compromised, it can allow essential cell materials to leak out or toxic materials to leak in. Think of it as a break in the insulation of an electric wire, a minute break in a gas line, or a tiny hole in a gas balloon. Any one of these situations might go unnoticed for a time but, if uncorrected, could have disastrous consequences later on. Or, worse, if it continues, its minor effects can accumulate and cause an entire system to break down.

Suppose the attack occurs in a place where the by-products of the free radical and oxidant can't be removed. For example, let's say it reacts in the lens of your eye or on the wall of a heart artery. Either case produces a damaged site that can grow and get larger. In a sense, the damage develops a life of its own and grows almost like a cancer. In fact, that's how heart disease develops. A damaged site in a blood vessel is covered and smoothed with a fatty material, called plaque, and it continues to grow.

By-products of free radical attack go unnoticed when they occur because they are so small. For example, your body consists of 50 trillion cells; if one is damaged, you'd never know it. In addition, each cell is composed of billions of atoms arranged in myriad chemical structures; if one is destroyed, you'd never feel it. However, if the damage goes unrepaired or continues to take place regularly, eventually it will accumulate and be noticed. Once the damage is obvious—for example, heart disease, cancer, or emphysema—it's almost too late to correct. That's why we say a free radical attack is insidious—you don't know it's taking place until it's accumulated to a very high level.

Many of our bad experiences are insidious. For instance, we get tired slowly and might not realize it until we're falling asleep at the wheel of our car; or we might be run down from overwork or heavy stress and all at once come down with a bad case of the flu. Free-radical effects are even more insidious than those obvious examples. Free-radical effects develop so slowly that we don't notice them until they are clearly evident. These effects include wrinkles, cancer, heart disease, cataracts, age spots, and others.

Suppose an oxide of nitrogen from cigarette or auto smoke interacts with something in our blood via a free-radical reaction and the nitrous oxide is converted to a nitrosamine that causes cancer. Suppose another free radical upsets the delicate oil in one of our cell membranes allowing the nitrosamine to enter the cell. That cell is set up to become cancerous. You'd never notice one cell out of 50 trillion, but let it reproduce every week or so for twenty years, and you have a sizable cancerous tumor. If you aren't carefully examined regularly, the cancer will go unnoticed until it's too late.

Suppose the free radicals from carbon monoxide in cigarettes, auto smoke, or city air react with a cell lining the wall of one of our heart arteries. The body responds by covering it with a smooth, waxy material—cholesterol—so the blood still flows smoothly. This is the beginning of the sludge on an artery wall, commonly called plaque, that causes heart disease. As the process continues, the sludge continues to build also. By defending itself with cholesterol, the body sows seeds of its own destruction. It's a short-term solution that has bad consequences in the long run. In the case of cholesterol deposits, they protect the artery in the short term, but, as they continue to build, clog the artery in the long run.

Or suppose the free radical damages one cell in the lens of your eye. Although it can't be seen, this single cell forms a damaged spot that scatters light and helps other free radicals form in the cells around it. Because it's only one cell—or even one hundred cells—you can't see the cataract until enough of these reactions have occurred. A doctor once described the insidious nature of cataracts like this: "When a conservative woman comes into my office wearing an overly bright dress, sometimes so bright it almost glows, I know she's got cataracts. Slowly, over the years, her vision has declined and she's never noticed, but simply buys brighter dresses to compensate for her declining vision. Once I operate and replace the lenses in her eyes, she'll ask herself how she could have ever bought such a garish dress."

Once cataracts are well established, the only solution is to operate and replace the eye lens. This now-routine operation usually restores vision completely. However, prevention is still the best medicine.

Each of these examples is important because it shows that they can lead to serious, often life-threatening illnesses, and each is insidious because it occurs at such a microscopic level and so slowly that it can't be seen, felt, or heard—not even for decades! Each example, though minor by itself, can produce the serious consequences of a blocked artery, cancer, or a cataract. Who needs to die early or put up with the hassle of cataract surgery?

ANTIOXIDANTS TO THE RESCUE

In over 4 billion years, nature has developed many ways to deal with free radicals and oxidizing agents. Let's look at the systems we humans have available for keeping oxidizing agents from smoke out of our bodies and for neutralizing them.

When nature chose to neutralize free radicals, it chose wisely. All the antioxidant materials in plants that protect photosynthesis—ripe fruit from going bad, oils from becoming rancid, and so on—are useful to all animals, including humans, that eat them.

We are still in the process of discovering antioxidants. We've learned that some nutrients, such as vitamins C and E, have a dual role in life. These nutrients are essential in the chemical processes that make up metabolism and also are effective as antioxidants. Scientists have established the Recommended Dietary Allowance (RDA, for short) of many nutrients the body needs as vitamins. These amounts are usually very small. The body needs much higher amounts of nutrients as antioxidants.

If an antioxidant is also a vitamin, it must serve two masters. As an antioxidant, it's sacrificed when it neutralizes an oxidizing agent. But as a vitamin in metabolism, it gets used over and over. Therefore, when we find antioxidants that also protect the vitamins, they have even greater potential for doing good. Think of all antioxidants as "protectors," and antioxidant vitamins as "protector vitamins." Vitamin C is an excellent example of the latter.

Our eyes are bathed with a fluid we call tears. Tears continually flush our eyes to remove irritants, such as smoke and fumes. But tears are active. They contain materials to kill germs and antioxidants to neutralize some oxidizing agents. There are antioxidants inside the eyes as well.

We all experience tears at work—at work to protect our eyes. On a windy day or in irritating fumes, our eyes often produce tears so profusely that they overflow and run down our cheeks. Some plants, such as onions, contain natural irritants named lachrymators because they cause us to produce tears. Police use this same defensive process to their advantage when they use tear gas.

Similar to our eyes, all mucus membranes including our lungs are bathed by a fluid that offers two forms of protection. First, these fluids—alveolar fluid in the lungs, mucus in the nasal passages, and saliva in our mouth—trap unwanted materials so they can be eliminated. Second, these fluids, contain antioxidants that neutralize some of the oxidizing agents.

On a cold day our nasal passages produce mucus so fast that our noses run. Because cold viruses thrive at low temperatures, this is the body's most direct strategy to get rid of them. Smoke and fumes also cause the nasal passages to produce more fluid to get rid of the fumes and to neutralize the toxins they contain. It's one reason why smokers often cough and blow their noses.

In addition to the fluids, our nasal passages are lined with minute hairs that literally trap particles and sort of "flick" them up and out. This process is similar to flicking a dust particle off your shirt or blouse. It's the basis of a sneeze, in which the whole system works in unison to get rid of some irritants.

ANTIOXIDANTS ALSO PROTECT NUTRIENTS

In 1524 Jacques Cartier, the French explorer, and his men had to spend the winter on their ship in what is now the St. Lawrence Seaway. Their only food was salt pork—no vegetables. Once winter set in, Cartier's men started coming down with scurvy, a vitamin C deficiency disease that, in those days, was fatal.

Friendly Indians showed Cartier how to brew a tea made from pine needles that alleviated and prevented scurvy. The tea saved Cartier and his men from disaster. The explorers survived the winter in good health and sailed back to France in the spring.

Until about 1985, scientists thought the tea prevented scurvy because it contained vitamin C. In the 1980s, Dr. Jacques Mescalier, who was searching for the components in red wine that reduce heart disease, reexamined Cartier's experience. He knew that the boiling water used to make tea destroys vitamin C and that pine needles don't contain any vitamin C in the first place.

Mescalier proved that a bioflavonoid, specifically called pyenogenol, in the needles was responsible for curing scurvy. This bioflavonoid is thirty to fifty times more effective as an antioxidant than vitamin C. About one gram of pyenogenol provides the same protection as fifty grams of vitamin C. Therefore, because the bioflavonoids react more readily with free radicals than vitamin C, they protect vitamin C from oxidation and spare even the most minute amount. Only 10 milligrams of vitamin C prevents scurvy under most conditions, but add the bioflavonoids, and even 10 milligrams of vitamin C might be a large excess. Possibly only 5 or fewer milligrams of vitamin C is required, and the men probably got that amount from other sources. Almost five hundred years later, we recognize that bioflavonoids are such effective antioxidants that they go ahead of vitamin C. We also realize now why people who drink a modest amount of red wine regularly are protected from heart disease. When it begins, heart disease is partly an unwanted oxidative process, and the bioflavonoids that start in the grapes and are passed into the wine act as a protector antioxidant.

Bioflavonoids are found in all fruits and vegetables. Citrus fruits are especially rich in them, especially in the white membranes in oranges, tangerines, and grapefruit. Their name comes from "bio," meaning biological in origin, plus "flavonoid," which refers to a member of a group of aromatic compounds. These compounds have a common chemical structure, called a flavine, which is an especially good antioxidant. This flavine structure is widely used in nature.

Until about 1990, most texts on nutrition recognized that bioflavonoids existed in foods, however, their antioxidant role went unnoticed. By 1990, our knowledge of free radicals and unwanted oxidative processes had reached a level where the value of all antioxidants, including bioflavonoids, was appreciated. Now bioflavonoids are seen as part of nature's antioxidant defense-strategy and are recognized as being on the vanguard of prevention. In fact, there are so many of them that it will be years before they're all understood. They are abundant in fruits and vegetables. Textbook authors are now giving bioflavonoids more recognition.

ANTIOXIDANTS REVERSE DAMAGE

Watch a major-league baseball game and you're bound to see players, often pitchers, with a cheek full of chewing tobacco. About 16 percent of major-league baseball players have precancerous gum lesions that can be traced to chewing tobacco. Oxidants and other materials in the chewing tobacco irritate the delicate tissues and the lesions develop. They start as displaced cells. Think of precancerous (dysplastic) lesions as a clump of cells on their way to becoming cancerous. In fact, you could think of them as more cancerous than normal.

In the early 1980s, research scientists suspected that the right antioxidants could neutralize the oxidizing agents in chewing tobacco and prevent the precancerous lesions.

They gave tobacco chewers (snuff dippers) either beta carotene, an antioxidant, or a placebo and told them to keep chewing. Beta carotene is found in any deeply colored vegetable, such as carrots and spinach. A placebo is a pill that looks like the real one, but contains inert material, such as starch.

About 25 milligrams of beta carotene daily reduced the formation of precancerous lesions by over 50 percent! Some precancerous cells, which form the nucleus of the lesions, actually became normal once again. This reversal of dysplastic cells implies a therapeutic process for beta carotene in addition to its preventive capacity.

If 16 percent of tobacco chewers develop precancerous lesions, and two or three carrots' worth of beta carotene daily reduces these lesions by over 50 percent to less than 8 percent, what would happen if these same people also got other antioxidants in similar quantities? No one knows the answer, but we do know that it couldn't hurt them and it might do more good. Or think of it this way: You get at least a 50 percent return on a very small investment.

AN ANTIOXIDANT RESERVOIR

The antioxidant level of our body is derived from the foods we eat. Some things we do, such as smoking, places we live, such as cities, who we have as parents (heredity), and many other aspects of our life-style can increase our need for antioxidants. These life-style factors seldom decrease the need for antioxidants. The size of our antioxidant reservoir and the eating habits that replenish it explain why some smokers don't get cancer; why some tobacco chewers and snuff dippers don't get mouth lesions; why some smokers have more wrinkled skin than others; and why some smokers are more likely to get cataracts. But most important, these findings give us something to focus on for dietary changes and food supplement plans.

We can draw another conclusion from Cartier's chronicle; that is, that we haven't identified all the antioxidants and the ways in which they work. Throughout the text I keep emphasizing food in addition to food supplements, because we still have to rely on food for most antioxidants, as many are still not recognized.

In fact, the whole concept of "antioxidants" is still emerging. We'll be identifying new antioxidants and how they work into the next century. Even after the chemists have identified them all, food will still be the most readily available source.

Smokers have special needs. Studies on vitamin C, the simplest of all antioxidants, indicate that people who smoke have much lower blood levels of vitamin C than nonsmokers. This finding supports two conclusions.

First, we know smoking contains oxidizing agents that are neutralized by vitamin C, causing the vitamin C to be destroyed in the process.

Second, we know from many surveys that smokers don't eat the correct amounts of fruits and vegetables, which means their blood levels of vitamin C will be low from diet alone.

It has been estimated that smokers need about *330 percent more* vitamin C to keep up with average folks who don't smoke. This is consistent with its front-line role as an antioxidant. However, keep in mind that what can be said for vitamin C holds true for all other antioxidants, such as beta carotene. Vitamin C gets our attention because it's a nutrient that is easily studied and widely known.

Later chapters will focus more directly on cancer, skin wrinkles, heart disease, and minor problems, such as cataracts. Each of these will bring to the fore specific preventive steps we can take. But for now, let's focus on immediate steps.

SHORING UP ANTIOXIDANT DEFENSES

Because antioxidants are obtained from food and food supplements, we have a tendency to think of our body as being passive and simply taking antioxidants from food for its defensive needs. It's not that way at all. We have a very active antioxidant capacity that is made stronger by eating the correct food.

Start Now on Antioxidants

- Eat deep green, dark red, orange, or yellow vegetables: three to five servings daily.
- Eat fruits with red, yellow, orange, or green flesh: three to five servings daily.
- If you're a coffee drinker, choose tea in place of coffee for one cup daily. If you can make a complete switch, evidence indicates tea is better than coffee.
- Drink colored fruit juices: real juice, such as orange, cranberry, melon, papaya, and the like.
- If you don't drink hot beverages, learn to drink iced tea made from loose tea, not instant tea.

Supplements

- Vitamin C: As much as 1,000 milligrams is good for someone who smokes. Make sure the supplement contains bioflavonoids.
- Beta carotene: Up to 25 milligrams daily, in addition to lots of colored vegetables.
- Vitamin E: 100 international units (IU) to 1,500 IU daily.

CHAPTER THREE

ANTIOXIDANTS IN FOOD
AND FOOD SUPPLEMENTS

How easy it would be if we could put all the antioxidants we need in a single daily capsule or drink. Unfortunately, that's not possible, because our antioxidant needs are extensive and ever changing, and there are too many antioxidants to deal with.

Science has discovered many characteristics about antioxidants. For example, while vitamin C is a single material, vitamin E consists of about eight variants. Because vitamins C and E are protected by bioflavonoids, it's important to get them together. Selecting the correct foods and food supplements calls for planning. This chapter will identify the major antioxidants, antioxidant foods, and a strategy that can be used for meal, snack, and supplement selection. But first let's learn about how nutrients are expressed.

RDAs: "RECOMMENDED DIETARY ALLOWANCES"

As mentioned, the Recommended Dietary Allowances (RDAs) have been established for many nutrients. Many packaged foods use the term U.S. Recommended Daily Allowances (U.S. RDA), which is a variation.

RDAs are revised every five to ten years by a committee of the National Academy of Sciences. After reviewing all the pertinent nutrition research, the committee revises the RDAs for all recognized nutrients and establishes RDAs for newly discovered ones. Nutrients that aren't as well defined by research get a "safe and effective" range designation. This range tells you how much is enough for good health and how much could be toxic to your system.

RDAs are designed to produce satisfactory health in the general population. "Satisfactory health" means freedom from symptoms that could be caused by too little of a nutrient. RDAs are related to age, sex, size, and activity levels; special RDAs are designated for pregnant and nursing women.

The U.S. RDAs, which are used to label packaged foods, are derived from the 1968 edition of the RDAs by the Food and Drug Administration as standards for nutritional labeling of foods. Because a label is limited in size, a single index was necessary and one was chosen to represent an average adult. So, if you read RDA in this book and see a number that is close but called a U.S. RDA on a food package or supplement bottle, don't be confused. Both RDAs and U.S. RDAs for adults are close enough to be considered the same.

RDAs Aren't Exact

Nutrition is not a precise science, and it is constantly changing. Further, the RDA committee builds in a safety factor to account for normal, human variation. Therefore, if I recommend that you take a 500 milligram vitamin C supplement, and you purchase a supplement that provides 400 or 600 milligrams, you're close enough. The same is true for all the other nutrients. However, if you smoke or live with a smoker, make your errors on the high side, because with very few exceptions, more of the nutrient is usually better.

Non–RDA Nutrients

In this book you will learn about antioxidants, essential oils, and dietary fiber, which you won't find on an RDA chart. These nutrients are at the cutting edge of nutrition knowledge and won't be given RDAs until enough is known about them as nutrients to give precise recommendations. However, all of these nutrients are internationally recognized by scientists and are essential for everyone, especially smokers.

VITAMIN C AND BIOFLAVONOIDS

Vitamin C is the simplest of all the nutrient antioxidants. Chemically, it's a single material named ascorbic acid, which comes from the word "ascorbutin," because it cured the disease scurvy. Scurvy is the result of a longstanding vitamin C deficiency. Today we see vitamin C as both a nutrient and an antioxidant that prevents many illnesses and slows aging. As an antioxidant, it helps prevent cancer, heart disease, skin wrinkles, and other cosmetic and health problems. Bioflavonoids found in most vitamin C–rich foods, such as fruits and vegetables, enhance the action of vitamin C and serve as antioxidants in their own right. In fact, many bioflavonoids are more effective antioxidants than vitamin C. In fact, they protect vitamin C.

Smokers can maintain the same vitamin C blood levels as nonsmokers if they get at least 200 milligrams daily. That's 330 percent of the 60 milligram RDA for nonsmokers. But there's more.

Recent research shows that nonsmokers need even more vitamin C as an antioxidant. The RDA focuses on vitamin C's role in metabolism and not as an antioxidant. Indeed, we need at least 300 milligrams daily as an antioxidant. So smokers need at least 500 milligrams daily, and probably 1,000 or more milligrams, the equivalent of five to ten oranges. Eating five oranges or their equivalent in other fruits daily would be difficult.

But that's not all. Heavy smokers need more vitamin C than light or moderate smokers. And as we age, our bodies need more vitamin C to keep its reservoirs at the same level. So, at about age sixty, we need approximately 50 percent more vitamin C than a younger person at age thirty. This adds up to over 1,500 milligrams of vitamin C daily for a sixty-year-old smoker. It's actually cheaper and more practical to get that much vitamin C from supplements than from food.

Table 3.1 lists the most vitamin C–rich foods. I've omitted acerola from the list; its fruit provides 1,644 milligrams per serving and its juice provides 3,800 milligrams per serv-

TABLE 3.1
FRUIT, VEGETABLE, AND JUICE SOURCES OF VITAMIN C
IN MILLIGRAMS (MG)

Fruits

25–45 mg	50–95 mg	100–200 mg
Breadfruit	Cantaloupe	Black currants
Carambola	Elderberries	Guava
Currants (red and white)	Jujube	Papaya
Gooseberries	Kiwi fruit	Pomelo
Grapefruit	Longans	
Honeydew melon	Lychees	
Lemon	Mango	
Mandarin orange	Mulberries	
Pitanga	Orange, navel	
Sapodilla	Orange, valencia	
Sapote	Strawberries	
Soursop	Sugar apple	
Tangerine		

Vegetables

25–45 mg	50–100 mg
Broccoli	Pepper (hot)
Brussels sprouts	Pepper, sweet green
Cassava	Pepper, sweet red
Cauliflower	
Collards	
Dock	
Kale	
Lotus root	
Onions	
Parsley	
Peas	
Seaweed (Nori)	
Swamp cabbage	
Sweet potato	

Fresh or Frozen Juices

25–45 mg	50–95 mg	100–200 mg
Pineapple	Grape	Cranberry
Tomato	Lime	Grapefruit
	Passionfruit	Lemon
	Tangerine	Orange
	V-8 juice	

Note: All food servings are ½ cup or 1 medium fruit or vegetable; all juice servings are 1 cup. All milligram values are rounded up.

ing. However, acerola is not commonly consumed. The likelihood of your eating foods that would supply 500 milligrams of vitamin C every day is very slim.

Therefore, use separate vitamin C supplements in addition to the basic supplement I recommended in Chapter 1. I strongly urge you to take 500 to 1,000 milligrams of vitamin C daily. Select a supplement that also contains 100 to 200 milligrams of bioflavonoids.

CAROTENOIDS AND BETA CAROTENE

Carotenoids are pigments found in all plants, where their roles are as varied as their colors. Over 865 carotenoids are known, and the list keeps growing. Carotenoids often impart color in bird's feathers, or even egg yolks, because the birds or chickens eat plants and grains; likewise for the flesh of some fish, such as trout and salmon. All carotenoids are antioxidants, but beta carotene is the most common carotenoid and is essential to green plants and humans. Beta carotene is found in all green plants, such as spinach, and orange and yellow plants, such as carrots and melons.

Beta carotene and a few other carotenoids are converted to vitamin A as our body's metabolic activity calls for it. About 6 milligrams of beta carotene daily serve our vitamin A needs. Any excess above 6 milligrams remains as beta carotene and increases our antioxidant reservoir. Most people's diets supply just about 6 milligrams of beta carotene daily, which is enough to meet the RDA for vitamin A but doesn't leave any left over for beta carotene's antioxidant protection. Evidence is mounting that 25 milligrams of beta carotene daily is a good protective level. Other research has proven that beta carotene is completely safe, even if you take enough to turn your skin orange.

Many epidemiological studies and direct clinical studies have confirmed the protective role of beta carotene. Indeed, all of the studies conducted on smokers or tobacco users have confirmed its protective role. Dr. K. Fred Gey and his colleagues at the University of Berne, Switzerland, pulled together all the information and concluded that a nonsmoking person needs 15 milligrams of beta carotene daily to achieve an optimum beta carotene reservoir.

Common sense dictates that a heavy smoker needs a higher intake level. In fact, direct studies on stomach and lung cancer in smokers helped Dr. Gey and his colleagues reach this conclusion. Therefore, in a larger study focusing on heart attack and stroke, Dr. Charles Hennikin and his colleagues at Harvard used 25 milligrams of beta carotene daily with outstanding results.

From these studies I conclude that a smoker, passive smoker, and people who work and commute in urban areas should strive for 20 milligrams of beta carotene daily; 25 milligrams would provide even better protection. It's definitely a case of "more is better." Table 3.2 lists foods rich in carotenoids.

A paper published in the journal *Nature* in 1980 by Dr. Bob Shekelle showed that heavy smokers who ate sufficient beta carotene–rich foods, such as dark-green and orange vegetables, had dramatically reduced rates of lung cancer. From this research he proved that beta carotene is protective. Following Shekelle's work, extensive research on beta carotene has led to the identification of the carotenoids' protective properties. Carotenoids seem to protect most those organs with exposed surfaces, such as the skin, lungs, eyes, aerodigestive tissues (the mouth and other tissues exposed both to food and air), intestines, and bladder.

Lycopene, a red carotenoid, seems to protect specifically against bladder cancer. The bladder is your body's toxic

TABLE 3.2
CAROTENOID-RICH FOODS
IN MILLIGRAMS (MG)
(PER ½-CUP SERVING)

Less than 2 mg	2–5 mg	Over 5 mg
	Vegetables	
Avocado	Beet greens	Carrots
Broccoli	Chickory	Lamb's-quarters
Cabbage	Collards	Pumpkin
Chard, Swiss	Dandelion greens	Spinach
Mustard greens	Dock	Sweet potato
Spring onions	Kale	
Swamp cabbage	Mustard spinach	
Tomato (red)	Peppers (sweet red)	
	Pokeberry	
	Seaweed (Nori)	
	Squash (hubbard)	
	Squash (winter)	
	Tomato paste	
	Turnip greens	
	Fruits	
Apricots	Cantaloupe	
Cherries	Mango	
Loquats	Papaya	
Mandarin orange	Persimmon	
Nectarine		
Peaches		
Prunes (10)		

waste dump and is exposed to many toxins. Lycopene illustrates an important point: You can't rely on beta carotene supplements alone for complete protection. You've got to eat a diet of foods rich in carotenoids and also use supplements. For example, tomatoes are red and, obviously, contain lycopene, but they're just so-so in beta carotene. Because smoking carries an increased risk of bladder cancer, it's worth having a daily plate of pasta with tomato sauce or a salad with tomatoes and red peppers. Or how about a wedge of watermelon for dessert?

In Chapter 14, I discuss how to use beta carotene supplements to improve poor skin color from smoking. For now, let's focus on a strategy that uses both beta carotene supplements and carotene-rich foods as antioxidants to prevent cancer, heart disease, emphysema, and cataracts. I'll start by discussing supplemental beta carotene.

As a smoker, your goal should be to take 25 milligrams of beta carotene supplements daily. Because that level will build a good antioxidant reserve and will even improve your complexion. (This latter advantage is explained later.)

To consume the proper amount of carotenoids:

- Eat four servings every day of deep green, yellow, or red vegetables selected from Table 3.2.
- Eat 4 servings daily to include deep green, dark red, or yellow.
- Eat the equivalent of ½ cup of tomatoes as sauce or cut up in a salad.
- Eat three servings daily of colored fruit, such as watermelon, cantaloupe, oranges, kiwi, strawberries, or other berries.

VITAMIN E

Unlike the numerous carotenoids, there are just four tocopherols, and four tocotrienols. These tocotrienols and tocopherals are known as alpha, beta, gamma, and delta. Not all of them metabolize in the body as vitamin E, but all of them are antioxidants. So, as an antioxidant, vitamin E is actually the collective capacity of 8 materials. "Tocopheryl" is an alternate spelling of "tocopherol," which is the standard form used.

Vitamin E is an oil that protects other oils from oxidation. Like all antioxidants, vitamin E is sacrificed to save other, more important materials. Vitamin E was never very plentiful in our diet, but now that we get by with fewer calories, smokers can't possibly get enough from their food. Because our need for vitamin E increases due to smoking and urban life, we must rely on supplements.

As proof of our need for vitamin E supplements, consider this: Research indicates that vitamin E protection calls for at least 50 IU (International Units) daily. Indeed, K. Fred Gey and his colleagues at Berne, Switzerland, concluded that 60 to 100 IU of vitamin E is required to build and maintain an adequate vitamin E antioxidant reservoir. Only two foods could supply that much vitamin E: wheat germ oil or wheat germ itself. Most people don't eat enough wheat germ regularly to reach that level. Supplements are the only answer.

We know that vitamin E protects against lung cancer, aerodigestive cancer, and emphysema—all problems related to smoking and air pollution. Studies of cataracts have given us even better information. In one study on vitamin E supplements and cataract formation, 400 IU of vitamin E daily reduced cataract formation by 60 percent. Research supporting these findings comes from many countries. Yet because we can't get over 50 IU from a normal diet, we must rely on food supplements.

Scientists have followed people for decades and, even for generations, taking blood samples and analyzing the levels of certain nutrients. They also keep frozen blood samples that have been taken from people who have died of various diseases, especially cancer, for comparison to new research findings. These studies leave no doubt that vitamin E protects against lung cancer and emphysema. Seen another way, people who have low levels of vitamin E are at greater risk of getting lung cancer and emphysema. Children of smokers aren't likely to get enough vitamin E to protect them. They also should take supplements.

Biochemists explain this disease relationship to vitamin E as follows: Vitamin E protects delicate oils that are essential parts of cell membranes and other tissue protectors, such as omega-3 oils, which are essential to nerve tissues and healthy metabolism. When these oils, tissues, and membranes are attacked by free radicals, the cells and tissues are damaged and made vulnerable to attack by other toxins. Vitamin E is an essential component of the fluids that bathe delicate tissues, such as the aerodigestive tissues, and especially of the alveolar fluid of the lungs. So vitamin E protects these tissues from the irritation effects of smoking. This protection extends to asthma attacks in people, especially children, who live with smokers or in cities. Not surprising, the children of smokers are more likely to develop asthma and emphysema.

The eyes benefit secondarily from vitamin E. It protects the lens from cataracts and the delicate oils in the retina from damage. It is the only antioxidant known to prevent nerve damage and stop age spots from forming.

ANOTHER LABELING DILEMMA

Vitamin E has been expressed as international units for most of this century. However, in the tenth edition of *Recommended Dietary Allowances,* published in 1989, vitamin E was instead measured in milligrams. For the dietary and supplement needs in this book, you can treat IU and milligrams of vitamin E as the same, even though the IU is a little higher. I will stick with IU throughout, as that is how vitamin E is listed on most supplements and processed foods.

We don't know everything there is to know about the protective effects of the tocopherols and tocotrienols. As antioxidants, we know they serve in many ways and in many parts of the body. For example, one tocopherol might work best in the aveolar tissue of the lung but not be able to enter some other tissue. Variety applies to supplements as well as food. A vitamin E supplement should contain a mixture of tocopherols and tocotrienols.

As mentioned, wheat germ and wheat germ oil are the richest and most practical sources of vitamin E. Adding wheat germ to foods, such as cereals and salads, is an excellent health practice. Similarly, vitamin E supplements should include wheat germ oil. How much vitamin E? Strive for at least 100 IU daily. Indeed, it's better for smokers and passive smokers, including children, to take 400 IU. Vitamin E is nontoxic and human use up to about 4,000 IU (about 3,000 milligrams) daily has been proven to be safe in rigorous, clinical research.

SELENIUM

Selenium, in contrast to the tocopherols and tocotrienols, is a trace mineral, meaning that we need very little of it. Selenium and vitamin E work together, which was unexpected because they are chemically completely different. However, it was learned that selenium and vitamin E have an equal ability to destroy free radicals, and they each work in different places in a living cell. A view of a living cell might help you see this.

Vitamin E and selenium are first-line antioxidants on the surface of each cell. As you move away from the location of each nutrient on the surface of the cell, their protective effects weaken. However, the region where the weak area of one overlaps with the weak area of the other is strongly protected. This overlapping area increases the protection of each nutrient beyond the boundaries you'd expect from each nutrient alone. Hence, the combined action of vitamin E and selenium is greater than either one's individual effect. The results are similar to two top athletes on the same team. The team performs far better as a whole than simply by the added proficiency of each individual, because one athlete's abilities enhances the abilities of the others and diminishes any weak points. A similar process prompts people to say a fine orchestra has a "sound" that surpasses the quality of the single performers.

We need very little selenium, and an excessive amount *can* be toxic. For example, the 1989 RDA for selenium is 70 micrograms (mcg). Smokers should strive for 50 to 100 percent more than the RDA. So, if you take 70 to 150 micrograms as a supplement, your diet will provide the excess. Seventy micrograms of selenium is so small that it would be a spec on the period at the end of this sentence. Now you see what we mean by the word "trace."

The best way to get enough selenium is to make sure your daily multivitamin-multimineral supplement contains 100 percent of the RDA. In addition to that, eat some of the selenium-rich foods listed on Table 3.3. Don't rush out and purchase selenium supplements thinking that if a little is

TABLE 3.3
FOOD SOURCES OF SELENIUM

Good Sources 5–15 mcg	Better Sources 20–45 mcg	Best Sources 50–100 mcg
Cereals, ½ cup	Finfish, 3.5 oz.	Egg noodles, ½ cup
Dairy products, 8 oz.	Meat, 3.5 oz.	Pasta, ½ cup
Eggs, 1 medium	Poultry, 3.5 oz.	Shellfish, 3.5 oz.
Vegetables, ½ cup	Rice, ½ cup	
White bread, 1 slice	Whole-wheat bread, 1 slice	

Note: Values cited are averages.

good, more must be better. That notion can lead to serious trouble. Keep your supplemental selenium to 150 micrograms, and you will not exceed any safety standards, even if your diet is rich in this mineral.

CRUCIFEROUS VEGETABLES: NATURE'S SPECIAL PROTECTORS

Eat your broccoli! Finish that cabbage! You need those Brussels sprouts! Sound familiar? Through the ages mothers have urged their families to eat these vegetables, and children have continually resisted them. That's how characters such as "Popeye" began. They were usually "heroes" invented to get children interested in vegetables.

Mothers' urgings were sound advice. Cruciferous vegetables are the oldest of all cultivated vegetables, and since the early Roman era, their health properties have been renowned. The link between cruciferous vegetables and smoking first appeared when scientists found that the risk of lung cancer in heavy smokers declined when they ate Brussels sprouts. Since the late 1970s, numerous studies on all types of cancer in smokers have verified this protective effect of cruciferous vegetables.

People who eat more cruciferous vegetables have less cancer, fewer serious problems with their digestive systems, such as ulcers, and better general health. These benefits are derived from the unique antioxidants in the cruciferous vegetables that, in turn, induce the body to upgrade its own defenses. So, as protective foods, crucifers work two ways: by providing antioxidants and by causing your body to build a stronger defense network.

Neutralizing some free radical producers we call superoxides calls for an enzyme named superoxide dismutase, or SOD. Superoxide dismutase disarms peroxides and superoxides. Cruciferous vegetables induce the body to make more SOD. SOD uses substances from cruciferous vegetables, such as indoles and phenols, among many others, to neutralize the free radicals. Think of SOD as a bomb disposal expert that uses the materials from cruciferous vegetables to neutralize the bomb.

So far, that's all good news. If you like cruciferous vegetables, which I've listed in Table 3.4, it's great news. If you like to get all your nutrition by supplements, you've got a problem. Supplements of the materials from cruciferous vegetables aren't available and probably will never be available. If you purchase cruciferous vegetable extracts, use lots of them, because the amount in one or two capsules can't make up for a serving of these vegetables. This is one case where more is definitely better, and there's no such thing as "too much."

TABLE 3.4
CRUCIFEROUS VEGETABLES

Broccoli	Japanese horseradish
Broccoflower	Kale
Brussels sprouts	Kohlrabi
Cabbage (red, white, and others)	Mustard
Cauliflower	Radish
Chinese cabbage (bok choy)	Rutabaga
Cress	Turnip
Horseradish	Watercress

As an incentive to eat more cruciferous vegetables, Table 3.5 lists the cancers they help prevent. As all these cancers are initiated by free radicals, it follows that cruciferous vegetables will help prevent cataracts, emphysema, asthma, age

TABLE 3.5
CANCER RISKS REDUCED BY CRUCIFEROUS VEGETABLES

Aerodigestive
Breast
Colorectal
Lung
Pancreatic
Prostate
Stomach

spots, wrinkles, and the other illnesses of aging that are accelerated by smoking and tobacco use because they also are initiated by free radicals. Indeed, many experts teach that aging is the accumulation of free-radical attacks.

GARLIC AND ONIONS

In 1550 B.C., the *Codex Ebers*, an Egyptian papyrus, laid out the therapeutic and preventive properties of garlic. Garlic was used in the ancient world as an antibacterial-antifungal, a vermifuge, a tumor preventive, and even to cure "hot blood." During World War I, garlic oil was one of the best materials we had for sterilizing open wounds. By the 1940s, antibiotics derived from molds were discovered and became more economical, so garlic fell into disuse. Ancient practices died quickly and became the material of folklore.

In 1944, while searching for antibiotics, Dr. Chester Cavalito, a scientist at the Roswell Park Memorial Institute, in Buffalo, New York, proved that garlic had real antibacterial and antiviral properties. In fact, garlic is better than penicillin at killing some bacteria (germs). For some fungal infections and viruses, garlic is still the treatment of choice. And garlic's antitumor properties have been proven effective and are currently being researched worldwide.

Onions, members of the same family, have many of garlic's properties, as well as one that garlic seems to lack: the ability to help prevent high blood-sugar levels. While the active substance that causes this hasn't been identified, the effects have been verified clinically.

We know today that garlic is an excellent source of unique antioxidants, and the same can be said for onions, leeks, shallots, and other edible bulbs. In addition, materials in garlic help modulate high blood pressure, or "hot blood," as the ancients called it. Besides, the antibacterial properties of these unique vegetables help us naturally fight infection and colds.

PUTTING ANTIOXIDANTS TOGETHER

Making antioxidants work for you requires a combination of good food selection and effective supplement use. Use the following lists of foods, and food supplements to guide your choice.

Food

- Fruits: At least three servings daily with one vitamin C–rich fruit eaten raw.
- Vegetables: At least three servings daily with one serving of a red or orange vegetable. Your selection should include a cruciferous vegetable, and more is better. (Remember to get seven servings of fruits and vegetables every day.)
- Grains and cereals: One serving of a cereal that contains wheat germ.
- Garlic, onions, and edible bulbs: Each day you should eat one of these in a salad or sauce, or as a condiment for another dish.

Supplements

- Vitamin C: At least 500 milligrams daily in a supplement that contains at least 100 milligrams of bioflavonoids.
- Beta carotene: At least 25 milligrams daily in a supplement.

- Vitamin E: At least 100 IU or more in a supplement that contains a mixture of tocopherols and tocotrienols in wheat germ oil.
- Cruciferous vegetable extract: If available, a freeze-dried extract of a mixture of cruciferous vegetables and garlic. More is better.

CHAPTER   FOUR

THE B-TEAM

D o you think that people either have cancer or don't?
If you answered yes, you're wrong. This chapter
provides you with an understanding of how cancer
starts and insight into how you can reduce your
risk. What's valid for cancer protection is also effective for
prevention of emphysema and other benign but equally degenerative side effects of smoking.

The 50 trillion body cells reproduce, on average, about
every seven weeks. So, in a sense, we're always about seven
weeks old, except for our brain cells and some others that
don't reproduce. Don't panic. We've got enough extra brain
cells to live over 150 years. When something goes wrong with
a cell's genetic material, it can become a cancer cell. Once
the cell becomes cancerous and continues to reproduce, cancer has started. If special "killer" cells of the immune system
don't recognize and kill the cancer cells, cancer has started
growing. After that, it's a job for the doctors who specialize
in oncology and surgery.

However, as mentioned earlier, there's an intermediate
stage when a cell is not normal but it's not a cancer cell
either. At this stage, medical scientists call it a precancerous
cell or, more scientifically, a dysplastic cell. Think of a ruler
that's labeled "normal" on one end and "cancer" on the other
end. The area in between the two extremes is the dysplastic
phase.

A cell can survive in this dysplastic phase for a long time.
A good example is intestinal polyps, which are clumps of

dysplastic cells on the inside lining of the large intestine. The longer the polyps are there, the more likely the cells in them will become cancerous. Scientists have learned that 2 percent of polyps become cancerous in five years, 24 percent in twenty years, with various levels in between. Similar statistics apply to polyps in other places, such as nasal passages and on vocal cords. Cancer is only certain when a clear diagnosis has been made. Up to that point, doctors can only speak of risk. So, the objective is to minimize risk.

A number of factors accelerate the rate at which a cell moves through the dysplastic phase to become cancerous. In the intestines, some major factors include a lack of dietary fiber, too much dietary fat, tobacco use, alcohol use, and not enough folic acid, a B vitamin.

We'll cover fiber in the next chapter, but for now I want to focus on folic acid.

THE FOLIAGE FACTOR:
FOLIC ACID

Folic acid is one of seven B vitamins. Its name comes from the source of its discovery—green leafy vegetables, such as spinach. When folic acid was first discovered, scientists called it the foliage factor. Once chemists identified it, the name folacin was used. Because folacin in its free form is an acid, it's also called folic acid. I prefer that term, because it refers to the active form, and some evidence now suggests that not everyone can convert folacin fast enough into its active form. Supplements usually contain folic acid.

Folic-acid deficiency is characterized by the famous "Popeye" cartoons. If you recall, Popeye would get weak, tired, lack energy, and become mentally confused. When he was in this state, his archrival Bluto could get the better of him, usually by stealing his girlfriend, Olive Oyl. But as soon as Popeye ate his spinach, his strength returned and he would "mop the floor" with Bluto. The cartoon gives a pretty good, if exaggerated, rendition of folic-acid deficiency and how easily it's corrected.

We no longer see serious folic-acid deficiencies like Popeye's sad state, even though our diet rarely supplies enough of this nutrient. Smokers' diets are especially lacking in it. Recently scientists discovered that, in some cases, a folic-acid shortfall can produce very serious problems, even though a person isn't deficient in this nutrient. A cell short in folic acid is more likely to become dysplastic. Shortfall means a diet doesn't provide the RDA in a particular nutrient. However, the shortfall is not large enough to cause deficiency symptoms. That's not surprising, because folic acid is required for correct cellular reproduction, and it works at the most basic level of all: where genetic material is manufactured.

Dysplastic cells that develop from folic-acid shortfall can cause birth defects during the first eight weeks of pregnancy. This is an especially sensitive phase during which very rapid growth occurs, especially of the face, spine, and brain. Women who are short of folic acid during the first eight weeks of pregnancy are more likely to deliver a child with a cleft lip, spinal deformity, or even serious brain deformity. But these same women do not lack enough in folic acid to be classified as having a deficiency. Recent findings suggest that these women don't convert the storage form, folacin, to the active form, folic acid, fast enough to meet the demands of early pregnancy. (See the Chapters 9 and 10 in to learn more about these findings.)

Armed with this knowledge of birth defects, scientists reasoned that a shortage of folic acid could cause dysplastic cells and increase the risk of cancer in adults. Scientists have confirmed that folic-acid shortfall accelerates the transition of cells in intestinal and other polyps to cancer cells. It probably occurs wherever there's a rapid cell growth. This observation was especially important for smokers and tobacco users. Oxidizing agents found in smoke, pollution, and even many medicines deplete folic acid. To make matters worse, smokers' diets are usually short on vegetables, and smokers don't eat enough folic-acid-rich foods to make up for the depletion. So, smoking works against them in two ways.

Smokers usually have some dysplastic cells on the lining of their bronchial tubes. They can be clumped into polyps on those tissues, similar to polyps on the intestines. Bronchial tubes start in the neck and continue to branch until they lead to the small bubbles, called alveoli, in the lungs.

In one study, scientists gave smokers folic-acid supplements. Within a reasonable period of time, fewer dysplastic cells were observed in their bronchial tubes and other aerodigestive tissues (tissues that are exposed to air and food). The longer the smokers took folic acid, the fewer dysplastic cells they had. The conclusion was clear: Folic acid helps reverse dysplasia in delicate bronchial tissues that is caused by smoking, airborne environmental pollutants, and other forms of irritants. Thus what occurs in one tissue, the intestines, apparently occurs in all tissues, just as we'd expect from basic cell biology.

In another study, scientists showed that if folic acid was depleted in the intestinal tissues, a higher rate of colorectal cancer was observed. Moreover, if the people who were likely to have depleted folic acid used folic-acid supplements, their colorectal cancer rate dropped by about 15 percent. Look at it another way. A few cents' worth of folic acid daily, less than the cost of a single cigarette, reduced cancer risk by 50 percent.

Now, pause a moment and recall what I said in Chapter 1 about the diets of smokers—not enough vegetables—and I identified a specific shortfall in, among other things, folic acid. Remember, we're not talking about a deficiency that produces symptoms like Popeye experienced. Smokers just don't achieve the RDA for folic acid and fall short most of the time. Think of it as always being a little behind. Unlike being behind on finances that you can cover, this shortage can spell serious trouble.

A smoker, folks who live with smokers, and those who chew tobacco should eat lots of spinach, broccoflower, and other good sources of folic acid. Broccoflower, often referred to as green cauliflower, is a new, genetically engineered vegetable that is especially rich in folic acid. Nowadays you can also take a folic-acid supplement with the other B vitamins. However, I'm not finished with the B-team yet, because you also need other members. I advocate supplements, but they should be balanced with all the B vitamins.

NIACIN—VITAMIN B₂

Until recently niacin was considered a "ho-hum" member of the B-vitamin group. Like all of the B vitamins, niacin was considered essential for good metabolism and important for general good health. Sometimes women, especially athletic ones, were advised to pay more attention to niacin because they often fell short of the RDA by 20 percent or more—not considered a deficiency. More niacin is called for when you're especially active; that's how it was discovered as lacking in the diets of female athletes.

However, now scientists have acknowledged that niacin has a special role that makes it anything but ho-hum. Niacin is an essential member of a system that repairs mistakes in our genetic material. This system, DNA polymerase, corrects mistakes in the very substance on which cell reproduction depends. While cell reproduction is still a metabolic function, it is more important than just running low on energy. No clear epidemiological relationship between niacin and cancer has been established yet—the research is still going on. However, some curious protective relationships have emerged. Dairy products and meat have shown a minor protective effect against cancer. As these are both good sources of niacin, we can speculate that, in the future, epidemiologists will clearly establish niacin's protective role as part of the basis for these findings. Because biochemists know exactly how the protective effect works, they can direct the epidemiologists more clearly.

With niacin, as with many nutrients, we've got a problem with names. The following names are used interchangeably for niacin: niacinamide, nicotinamide, nicotinic acid (no relation to nicotine), and niacin. For the purposes of this book, they're interchangeable, so just think "niacin" for all of them.

YOU NEED THE WHOLE B-TEAM

All B vitamins have essential roles in nutrition and health. Most of them are vitally involved in metabolism and the conversion of food chemicals into energy and into all our body tissues. Therefore, all the B vitamins are important for good health, energy, mental outlook, and tissue repair. A couple of members of the B-team (biotin and pantothenic acid) are also critical to the regeneration of some antioxidants. This metabolic function gives them a special role in protection.

Let's look at what the B complex of vitamins do, and then I'll explain why they're all especially important to you as a smoker, tobacco user, or someone who lives with a smoker. All of the B vitamins share common characteristics:

- They are essential for the release of energy from food.
- They are essential for the myriad chemical processes that take place in our body's cells.
- They are essential for maintenance of physical and mental fitness, healthy skin, hair, eyes, nerves, and all body tissues.
- The absence of any one for a long enough period of time can cause death.
- Most B vitamins are destroyed by processing, which includes heat, storing, and even light.

Table 4.1 lists the B complex of vitamins and the amounts required daily.

Do Smokers Need More B Vitamins than Average Folks?

Yes! Smokers are at greater risk for having dysplastic cells, so it's only prudent that they ingest more folic acid and niacin. However, smokers have a higher basal metabolic rate—BMR—than average folks. A higher BMR means that all the processes in the body are working at a higher rate than non-smokers. Since the B complex of vitamins are directly indexed to the BMR, it follows that smokers need more of them.

Indirect proof of this increased BMR comes from the observation that smokers, on average, weigh less than people who don't smoke. In making the comparison, scientists paired people by height, build, and life-style. Most important, they were paired by food consumption. Smokers weighed less because they burned more of their food calories. Seen

TABLE 4.1
B-COMPLEX VITAMINS

Vitamin	RDA
B_6	2.2 milligrams
B_{12}	3.0 micrograms
Biotin*	65.0 micrograms
Folic acid or folacin	400.0 micrograms
Niacin	19.0 milligrams
Pantothenic acid*	6.5 milligrams
Riboflavin (B_2)	1.7 milligrams
Thiamine (B_1)	1.5 milligrams

*No RDA is established in the 1989 listing; this amount is the middle of the safe and adequate range.

another way, smokers weighed less because more of their food calories were eliminated as carbon dioxide and water.

I speculate that a secondary reason for lower weight is that smokers' metabolisms are less efficient because their diets are more poorly balanced than average. Dietary balance is hard to study. Poor dietary balance means that some of the B-team of vitamins are in lesser quantity, with respect to the RDA, than others. Because these nutrients are required in proportion to the BMR, this imbalance makes for poorer metabolic efficiency. It carries a secondary danger, because the two B-team members likely to be shortest are folic acid and niacin, which are critical for preventing cancer and degenerative diseases.

Indirect evidence that smokers need more of the B-team vitamins comes from a study of smokers who quit and carefully maintained their prior eating habits. These ex-smokers put on weight even though they didn't change their eating habits. This carefully researched finding is direct proof that the BMR slows to normal after people quit smoking, so it follows that their BMR was higher when they smoked. The slower BMR means that the body is burning fewer calories to keep it working, and the extra calories are available for storage as fat. Our body doesn't waste extra energy; it stores it as fat for hard times.

Oral gratification is often invoked as a reason smokers gain weight when they quit. This concept teaches that smoking satisfies an oral craving that is made up with food. Though most experts discount this idea, there has been no research that proves or disapproves the theory.

MENTAL OUTLOOK

Forget the negative points of smoking and focus on one positive aspect: People who smoke generally have their spirits lifted, feel they have more energy, can concentrate better and even learn faster. These effects continue after the smoking habit is established, but they are usually no longer obvious to the smoker. All these positive points suggest that people who develop a smoking habit might have mild depression. In support of this hypothesis, people who try to quit smoking are much more successful if they take a strong antidepressant drug. In short, they substitute one mood elevator for another.

No serious clinical studies on mental health have been conducted to show that some people need more of the B complex of vitamins than others. However, indirect evidence suggests that the candidates for additional B-complex vitamins would be people who have mild depression—the same people who are likely to smoke. Add to those characteristics of smokers the fact that any shortfall in the B-complex vitamins shows up first in mental outlook as depression, confusion, and general slowness, and you make a secondary case for extra B-complex vitamins for smokers. That's why I recommend extra supplements. Use them sensibly and they have the potential to do a lot of good.

B-COMPLEX SUPPLEMENTS

I favor a general supplement that also supplies 100 percent of the U.S. RDA of the B-complex vitamins for average people. For smokers, tobacco chewers, and persons living with smokers, I recommend extra B complex. (This also applies to people who live in areas where the air quality is poor.) A few rules apply in the selection of a good B-complex supplement:

- All the B vitamins should be in the same ratio with respect to the RDA, except for folic acid. Folic acid should be at 100 percent of the RDA.
- The supplement should contain biotin and pantothenic acid within 50 percent of the levels shown on Table 4.1. Although they don't have U.S. RDAs, they are necessary for smokers.
- Each tablet or capsule should provide no more than 500 percent (five times) the U.S. RDA for all the B vitamins. If each tablet or capsule contains 100 percent of the U.S. RDA, it's fine.

CHAPTER FIVE

DIETARY FIBER NEEDS
OF SMOKERS

A daily balanced diet calls for five servings of fruits and vegetables, four of grains and cereals (including a fiber-rich cereal), and a liberal use of beans as a protein source. Smokers need seven servings of fruits and vegetables daily for a balanced diet. If your diet includes that much fruit and vegetables, and a fiber-rich cereal, you'll get about 30 grams of fiber daily, the amount various expert medical panels and the Food and Nutrition Board have recommended for average adults. Other medical panels have recommended an average of 40 grams daily. So, the consensus of expert opinion places an adult need at 30 or more grams of fiber daily. If you smoke, you should strive for at least 30 grams, and preferably 35 grams of fiber daily.

The diet of average Americans provides only about 12 grams of fiber daily; in other words, we get under half of what we need. Because we know that smokers tend to eat fewer vegetables than other people, we can correctly infer they get, on average, even less than 12 grams of fiber from their diet. That's more than a 60 percent shortfall! The consequences of getting less than 40 percent of the fiber needed are serious, and you'll never notice until it's too late.

Constipation is the clearest outcome of inadequate dietary fiber. Constipation can be defined as infrequent bowel movements—in other words, *not* having an easy bowel movement with soft, light-brown stools every twenty-four to thirty-six hours. Indirectly, constipation causes poor complexion, abdominal discomfort, digestive disorders, and several types of cancer. Constipation has been linked directly to many intestinal disorders, including ulcers, gallstones, diverticulosis, irritable bowel syndrome, colitis, hemorrhoids, varicose veins, and colorectal cancer. Smoking or any other tobacco use exaggerates the risk of each of these illnesses.

WHAT IS DIETARY FIBER?

Fiber is the indigestible material from plant foods, including cereals, grains, vegetables, and fruit.

The fiber these foods provide is different, but it can be classified either as soft or hard. Soft fiber is also called soluble fiber, and hard fiber is called insoluble fiber. Hard fiber increases stool bulk and produces regularity, while soft fiber increases the stool's water content and binds and removes toxic wastes. You need about three times more hard fiber than soft fiber. We'll use the general terms "soluble" and "insoluble" because they're more widely used on packaged foods.

All plant foods provide both soluble and insoluble fiber, but some plants are richer in one type versus another. For example, wheat bran is almost completely insoluble fiber, and apple pectin is almost entirely soluble fiber. You can purchase 100 percent wheat-bran cereals but are unlikely to eat apple pectin. However, fiber supplements sold in drugstores are likely to be 100 percent soluble fiber. A grain of wheat and an apple contain both types of fiber even though the wheat has more insoluble fiber and the apple has more soluble fiber. That's why people should eat a wide variety of plant foods and try to consume the recommended daily servings.

"Soluble" means that something, in this case, a food material, dissolves in water. For example, sugar is soluble; it will dissolve completely in water. Very few fiber supplements will do so. (Some guar gums and pectins will dissolve, but most of us never see them in pure form.) However, soluble fibers do dissolve more in water than do insoluble ones.

Table 5.1 lists the effects of fiber on stool volume and the ability of these fibers to lower cholesterol. Cholesterol-lowering ability refers to fiber's abilities to help detoxify our body. Hard fiber, such as from wheat bran, increases stool volume most, but all sources of fiber do so to some degree. By increasing stool volume you improve bowel regularity and move more water through your digestive system. Together these effects improve your health by helping rid your body of waste quickly. This means toxic wastes are in your system for a shorter time. Common sense tells us that's good.

| | | **Table 5.1** | |
| | | **Fiber Input: Stool Output** | |
Fiber Source	**Fiber Type**	**Stool Volume Increase per Unit of Fiber**	**Cholesterol-lowering Ability**
Wheat Bran, raw or cooked	Hard	5.7	None
Fruits and vegetables: carrots, cabbage, peas, apple, beans, etc.	Mixed	4.9	Fair
Oats: oat bran; rolled oats	More soft	3.9	Excellent
Gums and mucilages: psyllium, guar, sterculia	Soft	3.5	Excellent
Corn: corn bran, cornmeal	More soft	3.4	Good

Getting Adequate Fiber

Most nutrients can be short in our diet without us ever knowing we aren't getting enough. Even serious vitamin deficiencies usually don't show up for several months and then can be corrected quickly. Fiber is worse; when it's short, we become accustomed to not getting enough and not having regular bowel movements with firm, easily moved consistency. Or we take laxatives for uncomfortable constipation and think they solve the shortfall, when all they do is cover it up. A regular fiber shortfall—indeed, call it a chronic deficiency, as some experts do—shows up in twenty or more years as a serious bowel disorder, such as diverticulosis, some form of cancer, or a combination of both. Worse, the fiber shortfall can contribute to something as indirect from bowel movements as asthma or arthritis.

When you get adequate dietary fiber you will have a bowel movement every twenty-four to thirty-six hours. It will generally be light brown to beige in color, firm but not hard, and easy to move. If you get an optimum amount of fiber, you'll have the movement every twenty-four hours. In fact, once you get enough fiber you will probably become very regular and go at about the same time each day.

FIBER AND POLYPS

Chapter 4 taught that intestinal polyps are clumps of dysplastic cells with a high probability of becoming cancerous if a person has them long enough. A diet adequate in dietary fiber, especially about 30 percent insoluble fiber, prevents polyp formation. Moreover, some research indicates that the fiber actually helps make polyps disappear after they've formed. In short, they come and go with adequate fiber, but they come and stay with inadequate dietary fiber.

Now add to this knowledge the fact that smokers have a higher risk of intestinal (colorectal) cancer. It means that tars and materials that get into the system probably accelerate the transition of polyps to being cancerous. In my opinion, this should be a sufficient reason for smokers or tobacco users to switch to a high-fiber diet. The same goes for people who live and work in a smoky environment.

FIBER: NATURE'S DETOXIFIER

Dietary fiber, especially soluble fiber, binds unwanted material and helps the body detoxify itself. Many of these "toxins" are by-products of liver metabolism or of materials trapped by the liver. They pass into the intestinal tract through the bile duct. This duct connects the gall bladder, which is the liver's toxic waste dump, to the intestines. If these wastes aren't bound to dietary fiber, many of them get reabsorbed farther along in the digestive system. Then they can move via the blood and lymphatic systems to all parts of the body. Reabsorption of bile by-products is an example of nature's expectation that we will get enough fiber to remove them, and its efficiency in saving what we don't throw away.

We can use this natural ability to convert cholesterol to bile acids and thus to lower cholesterol by removing bile acids. Removing the bile acids is like removing cholesterol, because it causes the liver to convert cholesterol into bile acids and eliminate them. If they're eliminated, there's less cholesterol available to sludge up our arteries. Good cholesterol-lowering strategies are built around higher-fiber, especially soluble-fiber, low-fat diets. Oatmeal, beans, and some vegetable gums are especially good at lowering cholesterol. A successful cholesterol-lowering strategy also should rely on supplemental fiber, usually sold as psyllium hydrocolloid and labeled as fiber laxatives in drugstores and supermarkets.

Human clinical studies and animal experiments have verified the ability of fiber to remove both dietary and body-produced toxins. Constipated people cannot eliminate toxins efficiently because they have less bowel frequency and smaller stool volume than people who are not constipated and get enough fiber. Frequency and volume together produce the most efficient body waste removal. Consequently, constipated people have a higher risk of many illnesses, such as more frequent asthma attacks, heart disease, high blood pressure, most types of cancer, and intestinal disorders, among other illnesses.

Prevention is the best cure and merely calls for enough dietary fiber.

FIBER AND SMOKERS

Smoking increases the risk of many stomach and bowel disorders, but none are so ominous as pancreatic, stomach, and colorectal cancer. The risk of any one can be reduced with sufficient fiber. Following a good food and fiber-supplement program will increase your dietary fiber, improve your health, and remove several major risks from your life.

FIBER IN CEREALS

Any supermarket offers an array of cereals that make starting each day with a serving of high-fiber cereal easy. Table 5.2 lists fiber cereals that provide enough fiber to make them worthwhile. The list is by no means complete, because food products come and go. However, cereals with either "bran"

TABLE 5.2
FIBER CEREALS

Good Fiber 4–6 Grams	High Fiber 7–14 Grams
Bran Flakes	All Bran
Crunchy Bran	Fiber One
40% Bran Flakes	100% Bran
Fruitful Bran	
Fruit 'N Fibre	
Oat Bran	
Raisin Bran	
Shredded Wheat 'N Bran	
Wheatena (cooked cereal)	

or "fiber" in their name are usually acceptable. Read labels: A good fiber cereal will provide at least 4 grams of fiber; a high-fiber cereal will provide 7 or more grams of fiber.

FIBER IN FRUIT

Because fruit is easy to put on cereal, you can make your breakfast doubly good by topping a high-fiber cereal with fruit. Then, if you eat fruit for dessert and snacks during the rest of your day, you will be well on your way to a high-fiber diet. Table 5.3 lists fruits according to their fiber content. Snack on a pear, for example, and you'll be getting close to 20 percent of your daily fiber requirement.

FIBER IN VEGETABLES

A daily balanced diet calls for five servings of fruits and vegetables. For smokers, I can easily raise that to say nine or ten servings, but I compromised and set the base at seven. (See Chapter 17.) So, let's say you should strive for at least four servings of vegetables. In addition to providing a wealth of

TABLE 5.3
FRUIT SOURCES OF FIBER

Average Fiber 2–4 Grams	High Fiber 5–9 Grams
Apple (2 small)	Blackberries (1 cup)
Apricot (2 small)	Pear (1 medium)
Banana (1 medium)	Raspberries (1 cup)
Grapefruit (½)	
Orange (1 medium)	
Peach (1 medium)	
Pineapple (1 cup)	
Plum (3 small)	
Strawberries (1 cup)	

antioxidants, vegetables will add to your daily compliment of dietary fiber.

Table 5.4 lists vegetables according to their fiber content. Vegetables usually contain more soluble than insoluble fiber. Four servings daily will easily supply 30 to 50 percent of your fiber need. If you snack on carrots, for example, you can even do much better.

FIBER SUPPLEMENTS

In spite of your best efforts, you still might not eat enough fiber to guarantee the 30 grams of fiber you need. Therefore, you can use fiber supplements to push you over the top. One good thing about fiber is that research has shown it's just about impossible to get too much. Indeed, scientists have tested people at 90 grams daily and found no adverse effects. Therefore, don't worry about getting too much fiber if you use fiber supplements.

Table 5.5 lists a few sources of supplemental fiber available in most supermarkets, drugstores, health-food stores, or by direct sales. In general, the generic drugstore brands of fiber laxatives are excellent and cost effective.

To be practical, a fiber supplement needs to provide 3 grams of fiber in a convenient serving. The powdered fiber

TABLE 5.4
VEGETABLE SOURCES OF FIBER
(PER ½ CUP SERVING)

Average Fiber 2–3 Grams	High Fiber Over 4 Grams
Asparagus	Acorn squash
Beans, green	Beans, kidney
Beans, white	Beans, lima
Broccoflower	Beans, pinto
Broccoli	Brussels sprouts
Cabbage	Corn
Carrots	Peas
Cauliflower	
Eggplant	
Kale	
Onions	
Potato, sweet	
Potato, white	
Turnip	
Zucchini	

Note: Values vary according to variety, season, and location.

TABLE 5.5
FIBER SUPPLEMENTS

Product	Company	Type of Fiber
Daily Fiber Blend	Shaklee Corporation	Soluble/insoluble blend
Fiberall	Rydell Labs Inc.	Soluble
Metamucil	Procter & Gamble	Soluble
Vegetable Laxative	Generic store brand	Soluble

supplements listed on Table 5.5 are practical. They deliver over 3 grams of fiber per tablespoon and blend well in 8 ounces of water or juice. In contrast, fiber tablets are impractical because they usually call for chewing 10 or more tablets to get 3 grams of fiber and absolutely must be followed with 8 ounces of water, which often the directions don't specify.

Fiber wafers are somewhat practical. If they provide 3 grams of fiber in a convenient, easily eaten wafer, they're okay. However, it is absolutely essential to follow a wafer with 8 or more ounces of water. Fiber without water can cause serious constipation. That's why I do not encourage the use of fiber tablets or wafers.

BREADS AND BRAN MUFFINS

Most bread sold in our country supplies very little fiber. Indeed, I didn't provide a list of breads because high-fiber breads are usually local products. By purchasing breads made from whole grains and reading the nutritional panel, you can easily obtain 3 to 5 grams of fiber from two slices. That's 10 to 15 percent of your dietary fiber requirement. If you like to eat muffins, find a brand of packaged muffins or a recipe for bran muffins that contains at least 3 grams of fiber per muffin. Many so-called bran muffins are like the chicken soup factory where a resident chicken is dipped into each pot every day.

PUT FIBER TO WORK

Among Americans, a high-fiber diet is a misnomer; none of us is likely to consume a truly high-fiber level. As nations industrialize, the fiber content of their diet declines. In the preindustrialized United States and Europe of 1850, the average diet provided over 12 grams of fiber per 1,000 calories. In those days, women consumed over 2,000 calories and men over 3,000 and, on average, their diets provided about 25 to 40 grams of fiber. Many people probably ate diets with about 40 to 60 grams of fiber. In 1992, diets provide about 5 grams of fiber per 1,000 calories. Since the average woman maintains good body weight on less than 2,000 calories, and the average man on less than 2,500 calories, people don't come close to the 30 grams of fiber recommended. Indeed, a recent study showed that many people fall below 10 grams of fiber daily. In our society, where we get less than half the fiber our bodies need, a diet adequate in fiber is "high fiber" in relative terms. The return is more than worth the effort you invest in eating foods that supply adequate fiber. Use the food lists provided in this chapter and remember that along with fiber, you'll be getting vitamins, minerals, and antioxidants.

- Start every day with a good or high-fiber cereal topped with fruit.
- Eat four servings of fruit.
- Eat four servings of vegetables.
- Snack on fruits and vegetables.
- Use fiber supplements regularly. (See text for explanation.)

STROKE AND HEART ATTACK

A cut or scratch sets in motion a marvelous process we call a blood clot, which produces a scab where the injury occurred. The clot begins when specialized blood cells clump together to block the break in the integrity of the small blood vessels at the site of the wound. From the microscopic, blood-platelet standpoint, a minor scratch is like a large hole, so it takes a good-size clump of them to block the hole.

A blood clot is a complex process that begins with the clumping of platelets, and goes through many steps involving various specialized proteins, other blood cells, and even the mineral calcium. When a clot closes a scratch or cut, you're watching one of nature's most well-organized defensive processes at work. Surprisingly, strokes and most heart attacks result from the same process. But in strokes and heart attacks, the clot forms in the wrong place at the wrong time.

A stroke or a myocardial infarction—that's a heart attack caused by a clot, or another clump, blocking a blood vessel in the heart—begins in precisely the same way as the clot to close a scratch. Platelets clump together because of some disturbance and the process starts. If the clot blocks a vessel in the brain, it's a stroke; and if it blocks a vessel in the heart, it's a heart attack. An internal clot can happen at any age but usually, and, fortunately, doesn't happen before about age sixty. Among the several factors that increase the risk of stroke resulting from an internal clot, smoking tops the list.

Smoking tops the risk list because gases in smoke,

mostly carbon monoxide, make platelets more sticky and able to clump more easily. Scientifically speaking, carbon monoxide increases platelet adhesiveness and aggregation.

REDUCE HIGH BLOOD PRESSURE

Elevated blood pressure also increases platelet clumping—and therefore the risk of stroke and heart attack. Blood pressure is a product of the force with which your heart pushes blood through your blood vessels to get oxygen to all your tissues. Above-normal blood pressure increases the risk of stroke and heart attack for two reasons. First, elevated blood pressure makes the platelets and other blood cells stick together more strongly. Second, when a clump forms and a clot develops, it is pushed harder into the tiny vessel that it blocks. It follows that the higher the pressure, the harder the clot is forced into the blood vessel. These ill effects of high blood pressure are bad enough in themselves, but together they lead to more and larger clots.

Smoking also elevates blood pressure because the chemicals in smoke cause a slight constriction of blood vessels. This means that the vessels give stiffer-than-normal resistance to blood flow, so the heart responds with more force. We see the outcome as slightly elevated blood pressure. Consequently, one risk factor, smoking, increases the likelihood of developing the other risk factor, high blood pressure. However, because stroke and heart attack don't usually occur in young people, you might say: "Look, I'm only twenty-five or thirty years old; do I really need to worry about this now?"

My reply is yes! These risk factors accumulate with the years. That's the insidious nature of risk. You don't know your risk is increasing until you're sick or an examination prompts your doctor to give you a scare. You can do many things to reduce platelet aggregation and keep blood pressure in line. By doing them you will keep your risk of stroke and heart attack near to that of folks who don't smoke. In fact, if you exercise, you probably can bring your risk down to "average." Because you're not as likely as nonsmokers to be overweight, you've already eliminated one major risk factor.

Twenty-three percent of the population has inherited a

problem with keeping blood pressure in line; it is a definite problem for anyone who smokes. Over age sixty, about 75 percent of us get high blood pressure. High blood pressure is our single, greatest national disease, and everyone should take dietary and life-style steps to bring blood pressure into normal range. About 80 percent of high blood pressure can be controlled completely by diet and life-style. However, most people with high blood pressure use medication and not a diet. In the United States alone, blood pressure is a $17 billion industry.

Chapter 7 explains how to reduce high blood pressure by diet and exercise. If you've already got high blood pressure, or if you're at the high end of normal, there is much you can do to bring your blood pressure into line. If your blood pressure is still normal, prevention is the best medicine for you. Steps you can take to reduce platelet aggregation will reduce blood pressure naturally and help prevent high blood pressure. Start with vitamin-mineral balance, including calcium and magnesium (explained in Chapter 9) for prevention of osteoporosis. Dietary fiber also helps reduce blood pressure. By taking these preventive steps you will have started laying a good foundation. The major step to reduce platelet clumping, however, requires a shift in dietary oils. You've probably only heard of these oils, the omega-3 or marine oils, in passing. The name omega-3 oils describes the basis of their structure. Chemists assign the name omega-3 to these oils because all three of them have a unique structure at one end (omega means the end or last). Because of this structure, our body uses them in special ways. Because their major source is fish, we call them marine oils, although some plants provide them as well.

FISH IS BRAIN FOOD

No doubt you've heard the saying "fish is brain food." Although it's a ploy that most parents use to induce their children to eat fish, the statement is correct. The omega-3 oils we get from fish are used in brain tissue and in specialized tissues in the eye's retina, which is really an extension of brain tissue. But these same oils also help normalize platelet aggregation by reducing their tendency to clump. The omega-3 oils help to keep blood pressure in line in two ways. First, they reduce blood viscosity. (Viscosity is a scientific measure of the ease with which a fluid flows. High viscosity means it flows poorly; low viscosity means it flows easily.) The higher the viscosity of the blood, the higher the blood pressure required to move it around. So, if something reduces blood viscosity, it helps reduce blood pressure.

Second, one omega-3 oil is converted into a prostaglandin PGE-3. This particular prostaglandin helps counter the tendency of nicotine to cause small blood vessels to tighten up. This tendency to constrict, or "clamp down," helps to elevate blood pressure. Omega-3 oils also are essential to the function of our immune system and the modulation of inflammation. The former effect accounts for their influence on reduced cancer rates, and the latter effect makes them important therapeutically and preventively in rheumatoid arthritis, psoriasis, and even migraine headache.

Fish oils, like most essential nutrients, start as plant oils that accumulate best in cold-water fish. Small fish and sea mammals, such as whales, eat cold-water algae and plankton that contain an abundance of these marine oils. These oils are essential for fish and accumulate in the their flesh because omega-3 oils don't solidify at deep ocean temperatures. We suspect they also are essential for pressure regulation in the fish and mammals.

Even though most Americans eat few marine mammals, in some parts of the world these animals form a large part of the diet.

Where people eat an abundance of fish or sea mammals rich in the omega-3 oils, rates of high blood pressure, stroke, and heart attacks are much lower than they are in the United States. In addition to that, other diseases, especially inflammatory diseases, such as rheumatoid arthritis, are almost completely absent. Epidemiologists have confirmed these findings in clinical studies, so there's no longer any question of the value of omega-3 oils to human health.

The same oils are found in nuts, grasses, and a few other range plants. In the distant past, when our diet consisted of venison, rabbit, goat, and other free-range animals, we probably got much more of these oils from our diet than we do now. Indeed, nowadays a person must take special care to include lots of fish in the daily menus and use selected oils in cooking. In fact, the Smoker's Longevity Diet, discussed in Chapter 18, calls for four servings of fish weekly.

HOW MUCH DO YOU NEED?

We're just beginning to understand the need nonsmokers have for omega-3 oils, let alone smokers. But we can make an educated guess based on what we know. Dr. Kristian S. Bierve of Denmark, an expert on human need for omega-3 oils, recommends that the average person strive for about 1 gram daily of omega-3 oils as an optimal level. Though he and others haven't considered the needs of smokers, we can speculate that doubling his recommendation would be both safe and prudent. Safe, because much higher (about ten times) doses have been tested on people with no unwanted effects, and prudent, because the need to reduce clumping in smokers is much higher than in normal folks. I believe that 2 grams is appropriate for smokers, because their blood-platelet aggregation is nearly double that of nonsmokers. It follows that doubling the amount required would meet this elevated need head on.

HALF AN ASPIRIN A DAY HELPS

Since about 1955, various clinical studies on stroke and heart attack victims have suggested that a small amount of aspirin daily, about the amount in one-half tablet, reduced the risk of a second stroke or heart attack. Scientists correctly reasoned this was because the active ingredient in aspirin, acetylsalicylic acid, reduces the tendency of blood cells, especially platelets, to clump.

In the 1970s and 1980s, several studies were done on people who hadn't had a stroke or heart attack. People who were at risk for a stroke but had never had one were given a small amount of aspirin daily, the equivalent of about one-half an aspirin tablet, and were followed for five or more years to see if they had fewer strokes than people who were given a placebo. When all the results were in, it showed that the small amount of aspirin definitely reduced the likelihood of having a stroke or heart attack. Even though these results apply to people over about the age of forty-five, they are especially relevant to smokers.

Smokers of all ages have a higher risk of stroke and heart attack. As they get older, it follows that their risk increases more rapidly than nonsmokers. Therefore, the value of half an adult aspirin a day has special importance.

No, more aspirin isn't better! The minute I say that half an aspirin a day reduces the tendency of stroke or heart attack, someone decides to rush out and take more. It won't do any good. In fact, some evidence in these studies show that too much, say a few aspirin, can actually increase the tendency for stroke by other means. So more is definitely not better. Stick to half an aspirin a day and you'll get the right results.

A product that supplies 150 milligrams of aspirin is fine. Most adult products provide about 150 milligrams in half a tablet. Alternatively, you could take a baby aspirin daily and get the same result.

HEART DISEASE PREVENTION: A BONUS

Heart disease develops through a complex sequence that involves cholesterol and other blood fats. Smokers can reduce the risk of heart disease by increasing their use of the antioxidants (Chapter 3). However, the omega-3 oils (Chapter 6) add a special bonus.

There are two general types of cholesterol, the "good" and the "bad" cholesterol. In fact, the best index of heart disease development is to monitor the ratio of total cholesterol to the "good" or HDL cholesterol. HDL stands for high density lipoprotein, which is cholesterol that will be eliminated. Keeping the total cholesterol to HDL cholesterol ratio below 4 should be a national objective, along with keeping total cholesterol at 200 or less, and the lower the better.

Omega-3 oils help push the ratio in the correct direction by helping the body make more "good" cholesterol. Occasionally people who start using omega-3 oil supplements will find that total cholesterol increases. However, if they measure the ratio of total cholesterol to HDL cholesterol, they'll learn that their risk has, in fact, decreased. What happens is that some "bad" cholesterol is *shifted* to good, but more HDL cholesterol also was produced. Because all cholesterol is lumped into the total, the total can increase while the actual risk ratio decreases.

We will return to this topic when we cover exercise. Regular exercise is the most effective way to elevate "good" cholesterol. However, the best approach is to combine the use of omega-3 oils with exercise.

How Do I Get Omega-3 Oils?

We can make a three-pronged attack on increasing our omega-3 oils by eating fish, cooking with the correct oils, and using supplements. Each approach contributes to the total and can help you achieve the optimum level easily.

Table 6.1 lists readily available fish that are good sources

TABLE 6.1
FISH SOURCES OF OMEGA-3 OILS
(PER 3.5 OZ. SERVING)

Moderate 0.3–0.4 gram	High 0.5–1.0 gram
Bass	Anchovies
Catfish	Herring
Cod	Mackerel
Crustaceans (crab, lobster, shrimp)	Mollusks (clams, mussels, oysters, scallops, squid)
Halibut	Salmon
Perch	Swordfish
Snapper	Trout
Tuna	

Note: These values are relative. The best rule to follow is that the colder the water, the greater the omega-3 oil content. Fish rich in omega-3 oils usually are dark blue when viewed from the top.

of omega-3 oils. The variety of fish is sufficient to satisfy the most demanding tastes.

TABLE 6.2
DIETARY OILS RICH IN OMEGA-3 OILS

Cooking Oil	% Omega-3
Canola oil	10
Soybean oil	7
Supplemental Oils	**% Omega-3**
Cod liver oil	20
Flaxseed oil	57
Menhaden oil	23
Salmon oil	22

Table 6.2 lists the most readily available oils that are good sources of omega-3 oils. Canola and soybean oil can be used in cooking, baking, salad dressing, and wherever cooking oil is called for. The other oils on Table 6.2 should only be used as supplements.

TABLE 6.3
OMEGA-3 OIL SUPPLEMENTS

Product Name	Company	Capsules Necessary for 2 grams
EPA Marine-Oil Supplement	Shaklee	6
Max EPA	R. P. Shirer	6

Table 6.3 lists supplements that provide the easiest way to get omega-3 oils. A word of caution: Some fish oils have a "fishy" aftertaste. Although processing has minimized the problem, it doesn't alleviate it altogether.

OMEGA-3 OILS PUT TO WORK

- Eat fish four times weekly, and be sure to include fish high in omega-3 oil at least twice.

- Cook with canola or soybean oil and use them to make salad dressing.
- Add a tablespoon of flaxseed oil to your food daily, or take six capsules of marine oils daily.

HIGH BLOOD PRESSURE

High blood pressure is one of the most consistent health problems related to smoking. Research has never proven that smoking will cause high blood pressure in just any person, or whether the risk increases only in people who are predisposed because of their genetic history. Research has proven, however, that the blood pressure of some people with high blood pressure will usually return to normal when they stop smoking. So, if you've got high blood pressure, it's best to quit. But if you won't quit, read on.

Smokers can do a lot to keep their blood pressure in line and restore it to normal if it's out of line. This chapter will give you an excellent overview, but if you're serious about restoring it to normal, you must follow a complete dietary program. My award-winning book, *The High Blood Pressure Relief Diet*, available in paperback from Plume Books, explains every aspect of blood pressure control through diet. If you've got even borderline high blood pressure, I urge you to purchase a copy.

MEASURE YOUR PULSE

You're probably familiar with your pulse, but a quick refresher is helpful. Find your pulse on the underside of your wrist. It's on the outside as you look down while holding your palm up. I use the first three fingers of my left hand to find the pulse on my right wrist. Have someone show you if you can't seem to find your pulse. Use your wrist, because you'll be using your arm to measure your blood pressure. Some people use their neck to take their pulse, but you can't put a blood pressure cuff around your neck. Once you find your pulse, count it for a full minute. You're counting your heartbeat. Each time your heart beats it forces blood through your arteries to every part of your body. The pressure that is generated with each beat is the systolic pressure, and the remaining pressure between beats is the diastolic pressure. We'll get to them in a moment. For now, focus on your pulse. It should be less than 80 beats per minute and preferably 60 or less. If it's about 70, it's average.

Experiment with your pulse; take it when you're nervous, relaxed, after coffee, after a cigarette, and after climbing the stairs, and get a general feeling for how it changes. Your blood pressure can change similarly. Be sure that you or your doctor measures your blood pressure under the same conditions each time so you can compare the measurements accurately from one time to the next. The best way to take it is to sit and rest the elbow of the arm you'll be measuring the blood pressure in on a support mid-chest high. A table or desk is usually convenient.

BLOOD PRESSURE

Blood pressure is expressed as two numbers: diastolic and systolic. As mentioned, systolic pressure is the pressure exerted when your heart beats and forces the blood through the arteries. Diastolic pressure is the pressure that remains between heartbeats. Blood pressure is expressed as the ratio of these two numbers, with systolic over diastolic pressure. Both numbers are expressed in millimeters of mercury, and the systolic pressure should be about 40 millimeters higher than diastolic. For example, my blood pressure is usually 105 systolic and 65 diastolic. It's written as 105/65.

How Is It Measured?

Blood pressure is measured with a device called a sphygmomanometer. That's a big word for a simple device. The sphygmomanometer consists of three parts: the cuff, a device to detect sound, and a pressure sensor.

The cuff goes around your arm and gets pumped up so it stops the blood flow. The cuff is hooked to a column of mercury, or a pressure sensor, that shows the pressure inside the cuff. When checking your blood pressure, the doctor puts a stethoscope, or other listening device, just below the cuff to listen for the Korotkoff sounds, named after the doctor who first identified them. To hear them, the doctor slowly releases the cuff pressure and listens. At first, because the cuff is tight, nothing can be heard. After slowly releasing the cuff pressure, the first sound the doctor hears is "thump, thump, thump." This thumping is the heart pushing blood past the cuff with each beat, and the pressure then is the systolic pressure. Cuff pressure is allowed to fall just until thumps are replaced by a steady *whooshing* sound. Pressure at the instant the *whoosh* appears is the diastolic pressure.

Nowadays you can purchase electronic sphygmomanometers in drug stores and by mail order. Their cuff contains a sensitive listening device; all you need to do is pump up the cuff, and the instrument does the rest. In fact, some of them even pump up the cuff for you. Others are so sensitive that when you put your thumb into an orifice, the instrument does the rest. That's convenience and modern electronics working together.

These days measuring blood pressure has become nearly as easy as weighing yourself on the bathroom scale. New sphygmomanometers have a digital readout of diastolic, systolic, and pulse rate. Some of these instruments even tell you when the batteries in them are low.

What's Normal? What's High?

I believe that a diastolic blood pressure of 85 millimeters is too high. Systolic pressure rarely gets high by itself, but when it reaches 150 by itself, with diastolic below 90, it's too high. However, as on most other serious health issues, the surgeon general has set standards. I have summarized them in Table 7.1. These categories were established in 1984 by

TABLE 7.1
CLASSIFICATION OF HIGH BLOOD PRESSURE

Range in Millimeters of Mercury

Diastolic BP	*Category of High Blood Pressure*
Less than 85	Normal
85 to 89	High normal
90 to 104	Mild hypertension
105 to 114	Moderate hypertension
115 or higher	Severe hypertension

Systolic BP with Diastolic Less Than 90	*Category of High Blood Pressure*
Less than 140	Normal
140 to 159	Borderline isolated systolic hypertension
160 or more	Isolated systolic hypertension

the National Committee on High Blood Pressure and published in *Archives of Internal Medicine.*

High blood pressure is called hypertension, and someone with hypertension is referred to as a hypertensive person. As a practical matter, when diastolic blood pressure reaches 85 regularly, it is time to take action. A person with blood pressure at that level has a 10 percent greater risk of an early death than someone whose blood pressure is lower.

Hypertension is called the "silent killer" because most people don't know they have it until a doctor tells them. Its symptoms are so mild, and they usually develop so slowly, that it creeps up without the person knowing it. It's one of the world's most insidious diseases, because a person can be hypertensive and die from a stroke without even knowing there was a problem.

TWO TYPES OF HIGH BLOOD PRESSURE

Secondary Hypertension

Secondary hypertension, as the name implies, is a side effect of some other illness. For example, adrenal tumors cause high blood pressure; pregnancy sometimes causes it in women; some kidney disorders and other conditions also cause hypertension. Once the causative condition is corrected, the blood pressure returns to normal: for example, if the tumor is removed, the woman has her baby, or the kidney disease is cured. Secondary hypertension should be looked upon as temporary and curable. Only about 1 percent to 2 percent of the American population will ever get secondary hypertension, which accounts for about 5 percent of the total number of cases of high blood pressure.

Essential Hypertension

About 90 percent of all high blood pressure is called *essential* hypertension. It is caused by a number of environmental factors, including heredity, smoking, overweight, salt consumption, alcohol, and other dietary factors. All these factors, except for heredity, can be controlled. Heredity predisposes a person to hypertension, which they can usually avoid by controlling these environmental causes. In our society, about 23 percent of all adults have essential hypertension. It increases in percentage as people get older. About 4.5 percent of people up to age eighteen have hypertension. About 75 percent of people over age sixty-five have essential hypertension.

Eighty percent of people can control his or her essential hypertension completely. You must choose one of three courses. A lifetime of medication is one. Another is to follow the plan in *The High Blood Pressure Relief Diet* to control it without drugs. For a minority of people, medication is always necessary. The third choice is to accept medication and use diet to reduce the amount of medication to a minimum.

CAUSES OF ESSENTIAL HYPERTENSION

Heredity

Our parents and grandparents govern much of what happens to us in life. High blood pressure is no different. Many people inherit the tendency for high blood pressure, but by controlling their environment, they can avoid high blood pressure.

Like high blood pressure, people inherit the tendency to alcoholism and drug addiction. Some experts estimate that between 25 percent and 35 percent of us inherit these tendencies. However, most of us go through life without ever becoming alcoholics or addicts. Most folks don't succumb to addiction because they maintain control over their personal environment. High blood pressure is the same except most people have no concept of what they need to control in their environment. I'll explain what you can do as clearly as possible.

Overweight

Being overweight causes high blood pressure for two reasons. Each pound of fat requires about five miles of small blood vessels called capillaries. It follows that the heart must pump harder to push blood through these extra capillaries. Pushing harder means higher blood pressure. So your heart works harder if you are overweight.

Being overweight increases blood pressure for a second, more complex reason. Extra fat makes some people produce more of the hormone insulin. Insulin is absolutely necessary for the body to use the blood-sugar glucose. It helps transport glucose into each cell of the body. Overweight people produce excess insulin because their extra fat cells require more of it than the fat cells of other people. If insulin didn't have an affect on the kidneys, this would be okay; but excess insulin causes the kidneys to raise the blood pressure. Smoking adds to this insulin effect, so an overweight smoker has two problems.

If overweight people with high blood pressure lose weight and follow a diet like the low-sugar, high-carbohydrate diet described in Chapter 17, their high blood pressure usually disappears completely.

Salt

The K Factor

Most high blood pressure is caused by too much salt. Salt upsets a factor scientists call the K factor. The K factor is the ratio of potassium to sodium in the diet. It is very simple to calculate the K factor of your food. Corn has a K factor of 20 (219 milligrams of potassium and 11 milligrams of sodium), while corn flakes has a K factor of 0.07 (26 milligrams of potassium and 351 milligrams of sodium). Natural foods always have a K factor greater than 3 and usually above 6, while processed foods are usually less than 1. See Table 7.3 for more comparisons.

In a natural unprocessed diet, salt is very scarce. For example, in the early Roman Empire, soldiers were paid in a salt ration, much the same way early gold miners were paid with gold dust. The word "salary" is actually the contraction of "salt ration." In a few isolated places in the world, salt still has this value.

When the dietary K factor of a society is 3 or more, essential hypertension is very low—usually less than 2 percent of the population—and is mostly restricted to very overweight people. As the ratio approaches 1, however, high blood pressure in the population increases dramatically. Table 7.2 makes the point very clearly.

TABLE 7.2
HIGH BLOOD PRESSURE
IN A POPULATION

K Factor	Population with High Blood Pressure (%)	Hypertension Origin
3.0 or more	2	Secondary
1.1	26	Essential
0.4	33	Essential

Don't get the notion that the K factor can be restored by simply increasing the amount of potassium in the diet. It can't, because the total amount of salt—more specifically, sodium and chloride—must be considered. Most people with high blood pressure must control their sodium intake, salt consumption, *and* K factor. I'll give you some simple rules for this, but first, more explanation is necessary.

Sodium and potassium are the two major electrolytes in the body. A third electrolyte, chloride, is also essential. Electrolytes are minerals that we find in body fluids and tissues. Potassium is very plentiful in natural food, so consuming it in the correct amounts has never been a problem until the present era of processed food. In contrast, sodium and chloride are very scarce in natural foods. Our kidneys not only eliminate waste materials, they're also marvelously designed to conserve sodium and chloride, because, for about 3 million years of our existence, these elements were very scarce. In a natural environment, conserving sodium and chloride is one of the kidney's most important functions. So, not surprisingly, when there's excess sodium and chloride, which are the two elements in common salt, in the diet, the kidneys conserve it; after all, they've been doing it for eons. Through a complex series of interactions, this conservation of sodium and chloride causes an increase in blood volume, which produces high blood pressure. That's why we can't simply take potassium supplements to restore the K factor and expect blood pressure to become normal.

Salt Sensitivity

Some hypertensive people—about 50 percent, experts say—are sensitive to salt. These people cannot tolerate much more than about 300 milligrams of sodium daily, or about 500 milligrams of salt. By following *The High Blood Pressure Relief Diet*, these people can reduce their salt intake to 800 milligrams or less. If, after they do that, their blood pressure remains high, they will be able to get by with much less medication. By lowering their salt intake they will be doing everything they can to optimize their health. If medication can't be eliminated completely, reducing it to a minimum is the next best thing. The K factor and sodium and salt consumption must all be controlled.

Fiber will reduce high blood pressure a little all by itself.

However, fiber shortfall is not a primary cause of hypertension, as is overweight or too much salt. But studies have shown conclusively that increased fiber in the diet can help. Most people cannot get sufficient fiber by diet alone; they simply must use a fiber supplement.

Calcium-Magnesium

By a complicated set of circumstances, each living cell in our body must balance the ratio for sodium, chloride, potassium, calcium, and magnesium inside and outside. Research has demonstrated that calcium and magnesium are absolutely essential in this process. In some studies, all physicians did was provide selected volunteers with calcium-magnesium supplements, and their high blood pressure cleared up. I emphasize "selected," because these were people who had intakes of calcium and magnesium substantially below the RDA of 800 milligrams for calcium and 400 milligrams for magnesium. Restoration of these levels cleared their high blood pressure.

Omega-3 Fatty Acids

I call omega-3 lipid oils "nature's Teflon" when we talk of blood pressure. These oils are found in the membranes of the cells that line blood capillaries and the blood cells themselves. They have one simple but important function there: to make the arterial walls more slippery. They also make the membranes of blood cells, especially red cells, more flexible. By these actions the omega-3 lipid oils make blood flow more easily. Easier blood flow means the heart doesn't have to pump as hard to move the blood around.

How much of the omega-3 fatty acids are required? On a daily basis, I estimate that only about one to two grams of these oils is necessary if you eat a moderately low-fat diet. Follow the advice on preventing stroke discussed in Chapter 6.

Fat

Just as the correct oils help reduce blood pressure, the incorrect fat can help to increase blood pressure. Incorrect fat includes saturated fat. Processed meats are out, as well as high-fat cuts of any meat. Eliminate the skin of poultry and stop using high-fat spreads. Besides containing excess salt, they also contain too much of the wrong kind of fat.

Alcohol

Too much alcohol causes high blood pressure in most people, but some people are more sensitive to it than others. Alcohol makes high blood pressure worse for anyone, even if it's not the cause. It's worse because alcohol-related high blood pressure doesn't yield to medication.

The bottom line is clear: Hypertensive people must use alcohol sparingly, if at all. Some people shouldn't consume any alcohol. Not even one drink! For some others, a glass of wine, beer, or a mixed drink is the limit.

Fitness

Exercise will reduce blood pressure in most people all by itself. That's because most people are sedentary, and their vascular system is unfit. When they exercise, their blood vessels develop more flexibility and their blood pressure drops a little. More flexible arteries and veins mean that when the heart beats, blood is forced not into a rigid set of pipes but into an elastic and yielding system. The result is that lower pressure is required to get the blood where it's going. Look at it this way: It's as if the arteries help the blood along rather than resist its flow.

So, how much exercise is required to have an effect? Not as much as you think; about twenty to twenty-five minutes of jogging daily, or about forty to fifty minutes of brisk walking. There are many variations that range from swimming, skiing, rowing, or cycling, to a myriad of exercise devices. They can all be used. Read Chapter 12 on exercise for more information.

Type-A Behavior

Many books have been written on the emotional cause of blood pressure. None is as good as *Type-A Behavior and Your Heart* by Meyer Friedman and Ray H. Rosenman. This book teaches that there are some people who, by nature, are more tense, not relaxed, and live a life of internally generated stress.

One way that I can tell if a person has this type-A, unrelaxed personality is if he or she finishes other people's sentences. As a diagnostic tool, this test seems to work as a rule of thumb. These people can't wait for the other person to finish making a point; they must do it for them. If you are a type-A person, take steps to reduce the internal stress you generate.

External Stress

Stress is often generated externally in the workplace, the home, or even the neighborhood. You usually can't eliminate external stress, but if you don't take steps to reduce its impact, you can develop high blood pressure. There are two approaches: Deal with it and try to reduce it; or take personal steps to stop its impact on you.

Dealing with it requires a strategy that takes time and planning. I urge you to read *The High Blood Pressure Relief Diet* for some insights on dealing with stress. Reducing its impact on you is simple: Follow the diet and supplement plans in this book and exercise every day. Daily exercise, preferably at the end of the day, eliminates the ravages of stress on the body better than any medication ever can.

DIETARY WAYS TO DEFEAT HIGH BLOOD PRESSURE

There are four major ways to reduce high blood pressure: reduce your intake of salt and sodium; read ingredient lists and nutritional labels; and increase your water intake.

Salt and Sodium

- Do not eat a food that provides over 75 milligrams of sodium and any meal that provides over 200 milligrams of sodium. If you follow this rule, your diet will contain about 800 milligrams of sodium and much less than 2,000 milligrams of salt daily. Some foods, such as milk, contain natural sodium. These foods are generally all right because there's very little chloride.

Natural sodium still adds up, but it's not salt, sodium chloride, and the body tolerates it better.

- Eat for a K factor of at least three—the higher the better. With a few exceptions, you'll have to eliminate most processed food. Table 7.3 provides the sodium content, potassium content, and the K factor of selected food to illustrate how processing generally reduces their K factor. A glimpse at the table will show you why most processed food is out.

TABLE 7.3
THE NUTRITIONAL COST
OF FOOD PROCESSING
(PER SERVING)

Food	Sodium (mg)	Potassium (mg)	K Factor
Beef	44	311	7.00
Chicken breast	80	360	4.50
Corn (canned)	680	219	0.30
Corn (fresh)	11	219	20.00
Cornflakes	351	26	0.07
Fast food or frozen and breaded food	1,012	360	0.40
Hot dog (all beef)	461	71	0.15
Shredded Wheat (Nabisco)	6	150	25.00

Let's figure the K factor for beef. Most cuts provide about 44 milligrams of sodium and 311 milligrams of potassium; divide 311 by 44 to get a K factor of about 7. That's excellent. Now do the same for the "all-beef" hot-dog. Obviously "all beef" doesn't say "with lots of added salt." But look at the amount of sodium compared to potassium. Go down the list to corn. Fresh corn is great, but any processing does away with its greatness immediately. Canned corn illustrates another point: Canned vegetables are out!

However, there's a bright spot. Shredded Wheat is an example of processing without salt. Consequently, Shredded

Wheat is naturally low in sodium and has an excellent K factor. It illustrates another point: Read labels. Freezing doesn't alter the K factor.

Read Ingredient Lists

Reading ingredient lists is the only way to avoid sodium in processed food. If salt is listed don't select that food. Even if the product name or other labeling implies that it's low in salt, if salt appears in the ingredient list, don't eat the food. Recently the Food and Drug Administration caught a major canned-soup manufacturer for deceptive advertising. It advertised that its soups were good for the heart; but the government didn't buy its rhetoric. Although the soup was low in fat it contained too much salt, and high blood pressure is a major cause of heart disease. The label of the soups always show salt as an ingredient, even on the varieties that are supposedly low in sodium. Buyer beware: Read the ingredient list and the nutrition label!

READ NUTRITIONAL LABELS

Some processed foods are naturally low in sodium. In Table 7.3 I gave Shredded Wheat as an example but I could have included pasta as well. At the bottom of the nutritional label on processed and packaged foods is a listing of the sodium and potassium content of each serving. Divide potassium by sodium to get the K factor. Never eat a food that has a K factor of less than 3! If the nutrition label doesn't have the sodium and potassium content, and you have the slightest doubt, avoid the product. Vote for complete nutritional labeling with your money every time you shop.

WATER

Tap water and bottled water sometimes contain too much sodium. Often the sodium is found as salt, sodium chloride, in bottled water. Therefore, you must ask your municipal government about the salt content of your water. The label of bottled water should list the sodium content. Do some calculations. You should drink about 64 ounces of water daily—

in fact, I urge you to do so. That's two quarts. If the water doesn't supply more than 25 milligrams of sodium per quart, it's all right. Remember that you might not actually drink any water, but you get it as beverages and from cooking.

Water helps your body flush out the excess sodium and maintain correct fluid balance. Think of your body as a system of streams and rivers that are constantly bringing nutrients to your 50 trillion cells for nourishment. These cells produce any waste materials that must be flushed out through the kidneys and other excretory systems, including the sweat glands. The entire system requires water and works more efficiently when it gets the water it needs.

Ten Ways to Defeat High Blood Pressure

1. Sodium: less than 800 mg daily
   No food over 75 mg
   No meal over 200 mg
   No salt substitutes

2. K factor: at least 3; strive for 5
   Eat natural foods
   No processed foods
   At least 3,000 mg of potassium daily

3. Achieve ideal weight
   Follow diet in Chapter 17

4. Fiber: hard and soft
   30 grams minimum
   Daily fiber supplement

5. Water
   Pure water, 32 ounces minimum
   64-ounce optimum

6. Basic supplements
   Multivitamin, vitamin C, vitamin B complex, vitamin E

7. Calcium-magnesium
   800 mg calcium
   400 mg magnesium

8. Omega-3 oils
   Eat fish and supplement to get 1,000 mg daily

CHAPTER EIGHT

CONTROLLING CHOLESTEROL

AND HEART DISEASE

S moking increases the rate of what is variously called heart disease, coronary heart disease or cardiovascular disease, atherosclerosis, hardening of the arteries, and so on. It all adds up to the same thing: Smokers are more likely to die of a heart attack brought on by a blockage of one of the blood vessels in the heart. Blockage is the end result of having a buildup of sludge, called plaque, that narrows these blood vessels so that they can be blocked easily when an internal blood clot forms.

Smoking accelerates the accumulation of plaque by several processes. Materials in smoke irritate blood vessel linings and plaque is deposited as a protective substance. You can neutralize this irritant process by increasing your antioxidant reservoir.

For plaque to form, a type of cholesterol called "bad cholesterol" must be present. Its scientific name is low-density lipoprotein cholesterol, or LDL, for short. Bad cholesterol is neutralized by "good cholesterol" (high-density lipoprotein cholesterol, or HDL). The risk of heart disease is related to the ratio called a risk ratio, of total cholesterol to HDL, or good cholesterol. This risk ratio should be 4 or less; preferably less. Smoking increases total cholesterol and decreases HDL cholesterol, thus increasing this risk ratio. The higher your risk ratio, the more plaque you will accumulate on your arteries. Thus, smoking increases the relative amount of bad cholesterol and decreases the amount of good cholesterol. I said "relative" amounts of bad and good cholesterol because we want to lower total cholesterol and increase the amounts of good cholesterol. Do this consistently, and smokers can reduce their risk of heart disease to less than that of average folks.

LOWER TOTAL CHOLESTEROL

Blood cholesterol is accepted worldwide as the best indicator of the rate at which plaque is aging a person's arteries. Lower your blood cholesterol, keep it down, and you slow the aging of your arteries. Total cholesterol is easily and quickly measured by taking a small blood sample—just a little more than a pinprick. A complete analysis of the several types of cholesterol and blood fats calls for about a tablespoon of blood and requires a specialized laboratory.

MEASURING CHOLESTEROL

Cholesterol is measured as so many milligrams per 100 milliliters of blood. Since 100 milliliters is a tenth of a liter, it's called a deciliter. Hence, if there are so many milligrams in a deciliter, we can express it as milligrams percent. But generally we simply state the number of milligrams of cholesterol. For example, I usually say my cholesterol is 190, even though it's 190 milligrams per deciliter. When I say it's "190," people know what I mean.

C. Everett Koop, the U.S. Surgeon General under Ronald Reagan, declared 200 milligrams of cholesterol per deciliter as the number Americans should strive for. Actually, he gave the range of 180 to 220, with 200 as the target. Keep 200 in mind as your target and always try to beat it.

Other scientists want us to strive for a cholesterol level of 175 or less. They claim the 175 level is a sort of "cutoff" where plaque begins to dissolve off your arteries. They also claim we have to increase good cholesterol.

GOOD CHOLESTEROL/BAD CHOLESTEROL

Total cholesterol is a convenient number to work with, and the 200 target is good for most purposes. But, like everything else in life, we can become as complex with cholesterol as knowledge permits. If your cholesterol goes above 240 and you smoke, you'd better be concerned about "good" cholesterol.

We call HDL cholesterol "good" cholesterol, because it's an index of cholesterol that's being swept up off our arteries from plaque and dumped out through our excretory system. Therefore, we'd like the HDL fraction to be as high as it can go. Because there seems to be an average upper limit for HDL of about 60 for men and about 80 for women, we look at the ratio of good cholesterol to total cholesterol.

Good/Bad Ratios

Good cholesterol can be as much as 80 milligrams percent in women and about 60 milligrams percent in men. Therefore, if you're a man whose cholesterol is 200 and you have an HDL of 55, the ratio of total cholesterol to HDL cholesterol is 200/55, or 3.6; that's very good. In contrast, if your total is 250 and your HDL is still 55, your ratio is 250/55, or 4.5, which is average; however, at 4.5, you have a higher risk of plaque development than at 3.6. Table 8.1 lists cholesterol targets and risk factors associated with cholesterol ratios.

ACCURACY OF CHOLESTEROL MEASUREMENTS

Cholesterol measured in a lab is usually accurate to 5 percent. Cholesterol measured on the meter at your local drugstore or at a community health program can frequently be off by 10 to 15 percent.

So, if your cholesterol is 200 from a lab, the true results could be 210 or 190. If you have it measured at a community health check where everyone lines up, it could be reported as 180 or even 220. If it's within these limits, don't be concerned; just strive to lower it 10 percent. It can't hurt and will always do some good.

Your cholesterol level also varies naturally from day to day; even hour to hour, depending on diet, health, and other factors. You can eliminate most dietary variation by not

Table 8.1
Cholesterol Targets

Total Cholesterol	Heart Disease Risk
175 mg/dl or lower	Low
200 mg/dl	Average
200–239 mg/dl	Above average
Over 240 mg/dl	High

Ratio of Total/HDL Cholesterol

Ratio	Heart Disease Risk
3.0 or less	Very low
3.5	Low
4.0	Below average
4.5	Average
5.0	Above average
6.0 or over	High
7.0 or over	Very high

eating any food for twelve hours before having your cholesterol measured. It's also better to have a modest meal with no alcohol the night before.

However, cholesterol also varies by 5 percent with stress, exercise, sickness, smoking, your health, and other factors. So, if the true value is 200 and you just finished your income tax, it could measure in at 225. It will drop back to 200 in a few days once your nightmares about the IRS agent disappear. But some other event could throw it off at that time also.

The bottom line is this:

- If your total cholesterol is consistently within 5 percent of 200, keep doing what you are doing. Have your HDL measured and be sure it is enough to keep your ratio at 4.5 or lower.
- If your total cholesterol is 175, congratulate yourself and keep your HDL high enough to have a risk ratio of less than 4.0.

- If your cholesterol is above 225 and your ratio of total/ HDL is 4.5 or less, you're doing well. If it's above 4.5, start a program to lower your total cholesterol and elevate HDL.
- If your total cholesterol is 250 or above, take major steps to get your total cholesterol down and your HDL cholesterol up.

LDL Cholesterol

Another Risk Index

If your cholesterol is over 225 or if it's especially high, such as 250 or more, your doctor should do a more complex, blood-fat analysis. You will probably get an LDL, or bad cholesterol, analysis; some physicians and labs use it routinely, so I'll explain how it's used.

An LDL analysis takes into account the blood triglycerides. Though it sounds complicated, it isn't.

LDL risk determination is made from three numbers: total cholesterol, HDL cholesterol, and triglycerides. To obtain your LDL number, subtract from your total cholesterol your HDL cholesterol and your triglycerides divided by five (1/5 triglyceride). I make a good example; my total cholesterol is 190, my HDL is 57, and triglycerides are 95.

Formula: $\text{Total cholesterol} - \text{HDL} - \text{Triglycerides}/5 = \text{LDL Cholesterol}$

Jim Scala: $190 - 57 - 95/5 = 114$

Risk Classification for LDL Cholesterol

Less than 130	Desirable; the lower the better.
130 to 159	Borderline high-risk; take the steps in this chapter.
160	High risk; work with your doctor.

The equation teaches that it's most efficient to reduce total cholesterol and increase HDL cholesterol. It's even better to keep triglycerides within the 50 to 150 milligram range, even though 250 is still considered normal. Don't get the notion that grossly elevated triglycerides reduce risk, because they don't. Indeed, once triglycerides exceed 250, cholesterol seems to become elevated as well; when triglycerides reach 400, serious attention is required. Simply by lowering total cholesterol and raising HDL cholesterol, the triglycerides will usually take care of themselves.

WHY CHOLESTEROL GOES UP AND WHY IT COMES DOWN

About 80 percent of the cholesterol in your blood was manufactured in your liver. Cholesterol performs certain important functions and is used as raw material to make other body chemicals. So, our body needs some cholesterol; some experts place the basic need between 125 and 150 milligrams.

Bile Acids

Some cholesterol is converted to bile acids, which are essential for good digestion of fat or fatty materials. The gall bladder releases the bile acids through the bile duct into the small intestine just below the stomach. They combine with the food just after it leaves the stomach and help it mix completely. Bile acids are natural detergents our body makes to help us digest fat by mixing it with water. If we don't get enough of the correct type of dietary fiber and some calcium, bile acids get reabsorbed farther down the small intestine. Because the signals between reabsorbed bile acids and the liver are poor, the liver keeps making cholesterol and passes it into the blood instead of making more bile acids. So, removing bile acids with fiber and calcium is the same as getting rid of cholesterol.

Blood Fat

When we eat saturated fat, it enters our bloodstream through a complex, fat-circulation system called the lymphatic system. In the lymphatic system it forms into small droplets called chylomicrons. Cholesterol is essential to stabilize the fat that chylomicrons contain. Consequently, the more fat we eat, the more cholesterol we need in our blood. It's a natural fat stabilizer.

Experts keep pushing low-fat diets, because the more saturated fat we eat, the more cholesterol our livers must pump into our blood to maintain the right balance. Polyunsaturated fat (PUFA) doesn't have to be stabilized as much. We can tolerate much more PUFA, or vegetable fat, without affecting our cholesterol levels. In fact, cholesterol usually goes down when people increase their intake of PUFA and decrease their intake of saturated fat.

Excess simple sugar, such as the kind you get in "junk" foods, is converted to fat. Even though this fat is made in our body, it still requires cholesterol to be stabilized, because it enters our blood. That's why people who eat too much sugar have elevated cholesterol levels. The motto: Keep fat and sugar intake to a minimum.

Dietary Cholesterol

Dietary cholesterol elevates the body's total cholesterol level. However, unless you eat a lot of cholesterol-containing foods, dietary cholesterol will not have a major effect on your blood cholesterol. Generally, the same animal foods that contain too much fat also are rich in cholesterol. So cutting out one usually eliminates the other.

Abdominal Paunch

Overweight causes elevated cholesterol in men and women. However, men have a special problem with abdominal fat. Many men develop a paunch that seems to hang over their belts. Even a small paunch is enough to raise cholesterol. While a flat stomach looks good, it's also healthy. Smoking increases the tendency to have more abdominal fat. Therefore, smokers must watch their diet and exercise.

Abdominal fat seems to send a message to the liver that says: "Make more cholesterol." Deal with this problem directly by losing weight. Situps and exercises that produce strong abdominal muscles and reduce abdominal fat are especially useful to combat abdominal paunches.

FACTORS THAT LOWER TOTAL CHOLESTEROL

In summary, do the following things to lower your cholesterol:

- Increase dietary fiber. Soluble-fiber supplements lower cholesterol.
- Reduce total dietary fat, especially saturated fat. This means cutting way back on high-fat animal foods and increasing low-fat foods. Become more of a vegetarian.
- Reduce refined sugar consumption. Eat carbohydrates in the form of vegetables, fruit, natural fruit-juice, and whole-grain foods. Whole-grain foods include cereals, breads, pasta, and even some desserts.
- Get your weight and abdominal measurements where they should be. Men should have a waist-to-hips ratio of 0.9 and women, 0.8. This ratio is taken by measuring your waist and your hips, where you feel your bones, and dividing your waist measurement by that of your hips. As it exceeds these numbers, cholesterol creeps up.

ELEVATING HDL CHOLESTEROL

You also can reduce your total risk of heart disease by raising your HDL (good) cholesterol. If you raise good cholesterol while lowering total cholesterol, you gain a whole new lease on life. You reduce your total risk by 7 percent for every point you elevate HDL above 45. For example: a total cholesterol of 200 and an HDL of 44 yields a risk ratio of 4.5, which is good. Now consider a total cholesterol of 200 and an HDL of 50 with a risk ratio of 4.0, which is excellent. A small increase in HDL yields a significant risk reduction.

HDL is elevated by regular aerobic exercise; for example, by brisk walking for forty minutes, or jogging, cycling, or swimming for twenty minutes. Other forms of aerobic exercise, such as jumping rope, work as well. (Read Chapter 12.)

HDL also is elevated to some extent by increasing dietary PUFA and the omega-3 oils. This means eating lots of blue-skinned fish, such as salmon, mackerel, and tuna, and using an omega-3 oil supplement (described in Chapter 6).

HDL cholesterol increases when you consume enough soluble fiber. While soluble fiber decreases total cholesterol, it modestly elevates good cholesterol. It's like getting two effects for the price of one.

LOWERING CHOLESTEROL NATURALLY

In essence, you need to use a soluble-fiber supplement while increasing dietary fiber; lose weight, if necessary; reduce total fat and saturated fat; increase PUFA, including the omega-3 oils. That's a tall order. Let's consider how you might go about it.

Increase Fiber Intake

We need about 30 grams of fiber daily just to be healthy. However, as mentioned, most Americans get only about 12 grams of fiber daily from their diet. That's less than half of what we actually need. To consume enough fiber, we must eat a serving of cereal containing fiber, five servings of fruits and vegetables, and two servings of whole grains, such as whole-grain breads, corn, or wheat. Table 8.2 summarizes a daily dietary fiber plan.

Reduce Total Fat

Avoid processed and red meat and select low-fat versions of dairy products. Choose fish and white meats, and eat several vegetarian meals weekly.

Reduce Refined Sugar

Avoid highly processed foods, especially those that contain sugars or corn syrup in the ingredient list. Avoid sweet desserts, such as cakes, and learn to enjoy fruit.

Control Your Weight

Excess body weight results from too many calories coming in as food and not enough going out as exercise. Diet naturally by eating for bulk. A bulky diet rich in fruit, vegetables, grains, and beans provides eating satisfaction without calo-

---

TABLE 8.2
GET 30 GRAMS OF FIBER DAILY

Cereal (1 serving daily, with skim milk)

Choose from **soluble-fiber cereals**, including corn bran, oat bran, oatmeal, and psyllium cereal, or **hard-fiber cereals** (wheat bran), such as All Bran and Fiber One.

Vegetables and Fruits (7 servings daily)

Vegetable serving: 1 cup raw, ½ cup cooked, 1 potato. ½ cup cooked rice counts as ½ serving.
Fruit serving: 1 cup raw or ½ cup cooked, when appropriate. Or 1 medium-size piece of fruit, such as an apple, orange, or banana.
Beans: Include 1 cup of lima, kidney, pinto, etc. daily.

Grains (2 servings daily)

Grains: In addition to a high-fiber cereal, eat two grain servings daily. A serving consists of 2 slices whole-grain bread, ½ cup cooked corn oats or wheat.

---

ries. Burn more calories by establishing regular exercise habits. Exercise will also help shift fat to muscle and bring critical abdominal measurements in line.

Soluble-fiber Supplement

If you do nothing else, take a soluble-fiber supplement daily. Even with no other dietary changes, this supplement will reduce cholesterol. A soluble-fiber supplement usually consists of psyllium and is often called a fiber laxative. Soluble fiber eliminates bile acids, dietary cholesterol, and fat. Even people who eat a balanced diet generally don't get enough of these soluble gum fibers and pectin. These days our foods simply don't contain them.

When 3 to 5 grams of a soluble-fiber supplement is taken three times daily at meal time, cholesterol levels usually fall by 10 to 25 percent in one to three months. So, take a 5 gram serving of a fiber supplement before or during each meal, and within about one month, your total cholesterol will drop by about 8 to 10 percent. Stick with it regularly, and in three months it will continue to decline by another 10 percent, or more, if you also reduce your dietary fat. Be patient; your cholesterol got high over many years, so give it time to come down.

Lower Saturated Fat

Most saturated fats are obtained in meat and dairy products. You get them from red meat, processed meats, high-fat dairy products, and commercially deep-fat fried foods. So the easiest way to reduce saturated fat is to follow some food dos and don'ts.

Don't Eat

- Red meat, including beef, pork, lamb, and the like, more than once weekly.
- Processed meat of any type, including those made from turkey or chicken. (Surprisingly, these are often higher in fat than those made from beef.)
- Organ meat, including liver, kidney, brains, heart, stomach, and the like.
- Poultry skin.
- Fried foods, including deep-fat fried fish.
- High-fat dairy products, including milk, butter, cheese, ice cream, and yogurt.

Do Eat

- White meat of poultry with skin removed.
- Fish, including shellfish (four times weekly or more).
- Water fowl with skin removed.
- Low-fat dairy products, including milk, ice cream, and yogurt; cottage, ricotta, mozzarella, and other low-fat cheeses.
- Corn oil margarine.

Exercise

Exercise helps lower total cholesterol and is essential to raise HDL cholesterol. Exercise should be part of the total, risk-reduction program.

Niacin: An Aggressive
Cholesterol-Lowering Approach

Studies have shown that niacin, one of the B vitamins, can profoundly lower cholesterol and reduce heart disease risk. Niacin brings on several important changes in some people:

- It reduces triglycerides.
- It reduces production of the fraction of cholesterol that goes into the LDL determination.
- It elevates HDL cholesterol and reduces risk.
- It lowers total cholesterol.

Therefore, if you add niacin while you follow the program outlined in this book, you will reduce your risk of heart disease even more. That's the good news. The bad news is that we're dealing with therapeutic amounts of a vitamin; in effect, it becomes a drug, and you should consult with your doctor.

How Much Niacin

Some physicians have used from 3 to 8 grams of niacin daily with spectacular results. However, this use of niacin is the realm of medicine. Niacin's side effects—flushing of the face, nausea, itching, and others—can be very uncomfortable but not serious. Many people have been very successful taking levels of only 1 gram daily, which usually doesn't have noticeable side effects.

People start with 250 milligrams of niacin and work up to four 250 milligrams tablets daily over a period of about two months. At this 1 gram level, niacin causes about a 10 percent reduction in total cholesterol and a similar elevation of HDL cholesterol. It takes about six months for the effects of niacin to emerge fully. Add this supplemental use of niacin to a fiber-supplement plan with exercise, and you can gain a 25 percent cholesterol reduction.

If your total cholesterol is above 250 or your HDL cholesterol is very low, follow the soluble-fiber plan in this book and ask your physician if you also can try niacin therapy. Compared to other drugs, niacin is inexpensive. Its side effects aren't bad—many people have none—and usually diminish over time.

Prescription Drugs

A number of other prescription drugs are prescribed routinely to lower cholesterol and elevate HDL (good) cholesterol. They are resins that act like a super type of fiber and are generally used when diet doesn't have an effect or when total cholesterol is over 300. When people have such high cholesterol, most times a medical condition is causing it, despite whatever diet the patient follows. Medication to reduce risk is the only course to follow.

CHAPTER NINE

BUILDING STRONG BONES

A ll women have a risk of developing osteoporosis as they age. Women who smoke or live with a smoker have a much higher than average risk of developing osteoporosis. Osteoporosis means exactly what its name implies: *osteo* means "bones"; *porosis* means "porous." Osteoporosis accelerated by smoking is another one of those insidious diseases that sneak up over about twenty-five years or more, and seem to emerge all at once. Osteoporosis affects most women and very few men. Prevention of osteoporosis is not only the best medicine, it's the only medicine.

A BRIEF HISTORY OF POROUS BONES

Osteoporosis is a disease in which the bones lose calcium and become porous. An osteoporotic bone is more like brittle, plastic foam with its myriad small bubbles of air, than a stiff, solid, plastic block. A normal bone is hard and dense, while an osteoporotic bone is spongy, light, and very brittle.

Calcium is a dynamic bone mineral. Your blood calcium is always about 10 milligrams per 100 milliliters of blood, give or take 1 milligram. In lay terms, it's often referred to as 10 milligrams percent, or sometimes people simply say "a calcium count of 10." People always lose some calcium in urine, sweat, and stools, even if they don't get any calcium in the diet at all. It's a little like a bank account where there's always some cash outflow, whether or not there's some cash input. However, under conditions of all loss and no gain, called negative calcium balance, a person's blood level would always chug along at about 10 milligrams percent. How can the blood level stay the same if you eat no calcium and lose some daily?

Simple. People have an incredible calcium reservoir in the body disguised as bones. If you get more calcium than you lose—maintain positive balance—and do other things right, such as exercise, your bones build a little calcium and stay dense. If you excrete more calcium than you eat, your bones lose a little. That's why we say calcium is dynamic, because it's constantly coming and going, but the blood level remains practically constant. Your blood level of calcium is so stable that a departure from the normal range is cause for serious concern. Indeed, if your blood calcium departs from normal, your doctor will investigate to learn why.

Beginning at about age fifteen, most young women usually stop getting enough dietary calcium regularly. This means they are in a state of negative calcium balance, on average, and they lose a little more calcium than their diet supplies. This deficit is usually small, so it goes unnoticed. The backbone is probably most vulnerable to the loss, but other bones—for example, the hips, often the ankles and lower jawbone—seem to be a little more vulnerable, in that order. The backbone and the bone on which the bottom teeth reside are naturally "spongy," shock-absorbing bones. This seems to predispose them to lose their calcium first.

As menopause approaches, a woman slows her production of estrogen. Estrogen, a hormone produced by women, is necessary to activate bone cells that deposit calcium. Once women go through menopause and estrogen production slows to a trickle or stops completely, bone loss accelerates unless they eat enough dietary calcium and exercise consistently. Sometimes supplemental calcium isn't enough, and additional estrogen is necessary.

Estrogen is prescribed when a woman has definite bone loss or one of the major risks, which include smoking or passive smoking, inherited risk (female relatives with osteoporosis), high coffee use, high meat consumption, light skin and hair, and blue eyes. Additionally, residing in a metropolitan area with unclean air also increases calcium loss. But even with estrogen and calcium, a few life-style activities, such as exercise and moderate coffee use, are essential to keep bones healthy. Aside from the normal effects of aging, smoking, living with a smoker, or residing in a metropolitan area increases the rate of calcium loss.

Women who smoke (passive and active) don't produce as much estrogen as nonsmoking women. This nicotine-caused estrogen decline slows bone building if there's adequate dietary calcium and accelerates bone loss if there's inadequate dietary calcium. But even if bone loss accelerates a little, you still won't notice the loss, because the bones represent such a large reservoir. That's why osteoporosis is an insidious disease.

Think through the math with me for a moment. If you had a net loss of 5 milligrams of calcium a day starting at about age twenty, that would come to 350 grams of calcium lost by age forty. That's just over three-fourths of a pound. A woman weighing 120 at age forty should contain about five pounds of calcium in her bones. If she's lost three-fourths of a pound, she's 15 percent short! Yet all those years her blood calcium chugged along at 10 milligrams percent. You might ask: How will this shortfall show up? It won't, except by very sophisticated radiological measurements ordered by a doctor.

As a woman approaches menopause between age forty-five and fifty-five, estrogen production slows down and the calcium loss accelerates. Because the backbone gives up calcium first, her shoulders start to round a little, and she might notice some low-back pain. An aspirin will fix the pain. As this bone loss continues, she will actually become shorter. If the calcium loss becomes severe, she could develop several crushed vertebrate (bones in the back) and, by age sixty-five or seventy, could be up to six inches shorter than she was at age thirty. Add the slight "hump" that comes with this calcium loss, and you've got the little old lady with the dowager's hump. We used to think of it as "aging." In a sense, the dowager's hump shows the aging process at work, but now we can put an end to that kind of aging, even if you smoke!

A main argument in favor of building and maintaining strong bones is the prevention of shattered bones. Osteoporotic bones are more fragile than solid, dense bones. Osteoporotic bones don't break like a stick; they shatter like glass. Which one could a doctor repair more easily: the shattered glass or the broken stick?

Epidemiologists have proven that once an older woman shatters a bone, she's likely to die within the year. And that year might be spent in a wheelchair. This rather grim picture will happen to you only if you let it. Osteoporosis doesn't need to develop even if you smoke three packs a day. All you've got to do is make your body keep your bones dense.

How to Build and Keep Dense Bones

First, you've got to get enough calcium. This means getting at least 1,000 milligrams daily for all women past the teenage years. Some experts argue in favor of 1,200 milligrams daily. Indeed, others recommend 1,500 to 2,000 milligrams daily. You need this much calcium because your body only absorbs about 40 percent of the calcium you eat, no matter what food or food supplement it's in. But nature doesn't waste the extra calcium, because it plays a role in reducing heart disease and the risk of colonic cancer.

A smoker should strive for 1,200 milligrams of calcium daily; 1,500 milligrams is even better. Regular weight-bearing exercise makes dietary calcium more effective. We'll touch on exercise again in this chapter and extensively in Chapter 12. Magnesium is a second mineral that's also essential for good health and seldom gets the recognition it deserves. Magnesium works closely with calcium and is found in many of the same foods. Strive for 400 milligrams of magnesium daily.

The best sources of calcium are dairy products. Table 9.1 lists the best calcium sources. Peruse the table and you'll see that diet isn't likely to get you there unless you really like dairy products. Some calcium-rich vegetables also contain plant acids that make the calcium difficult for our body to use.

Look at the number of servings necessary to obtain 1,000 milligrams of calcium and you'll realize that low-fat dairy products are essential if you don't want to use supplements. That gets us to Table 9.2: I've listed the composition of an ideal calcium supplement. This information, or something

TABLE 9.1
PRACTICAL CALCIUM FOOD SOURCES

Food	Serving	Food Calcium	Servings for 1,000 mg
Sardines, with bones	3 oz.	372	2.6
2% milk	1 cup	352	2.8
Skim milk	1 cup	296	3.4
Yogurt (low-fat)	1 cup	272	3.7
Oysters	¾ cup	170	5.9
Canned salmon, with bones	3 oz.	167	6.0
Collard greens	½ cup	145	6.8
Spinach	½ cup	106	9.4
Creamed cottage cheese	¼ cup	58	17.3
Broccoli	½ cup	49	20.0
Beans	½ cup	45	22.0

close to it, should appear on the right-hand panel of the supplement label.

Notice this supplement contains magnesium, which is a mineral that works with calcium and is usually deficient in the American diet. Magnesium is essential for energy, bone development, maintaining normal blood pressure, and good nerve function. Your diet and a general multivitamin-multimineral supplement should provide from 800 to 1,000 milligrams of calcium daily. By using from one to four tablets of the calcium supplement on Table 9.2, you could raise your daily calcium level up to 2,000 milligrams.

EXERCISE AND BONE

"If you don't use it, you lose it" is an old saying that applies to everything we have, but especially our bones. It takes energy for your body to maintain strong, dense bones. Consequently, if you don't use your bones, your brain's most primitive logic says: Relax, let go of some of that calcium.

Bone loss starts as soon as astronauts enter the weight-

TABLE 9.2
A GOOD CALCIUM SUPPLEMENT

Four tablets supply:

Minerals	Milligrams	Percent of RDA
Calcium	1,000	100
Phosphorus	500	50
Magnesium	400	100
Optional:˜		
Vitamin D	200 IU	50

lessness of space. The primitive signal in their brain says: Let go. It's the body trying to be as efficient as possible. The astronauts combat this loss in two ways: They take calcium, and they exercise. Exercise sends a countersignal to the brain that says: I need the bones; look at all this work I'm doing. The fact that astronauts really can't exercise enough in space to overcome the bone loss is a major physiological problem of space travel, and much research is directed at its solution.

I used the weightlessness of space to illustrate how willingly the body lets go of its bone calcium. It confirms that the body must spend energy to maintain strong bones and that if we don't use them regularly, they simply lose their calcium and become weak. Therefore, in addition to providing enough calcium, you've got to exercise as well.

So you ask, "What exercise and how often?" Weight-bearing exercise is the best and most effective if done four or five times weekly. A brisk walk while carrying hand weights is excellent. The important thing is to walk for at least thirty minutes and, ideally, about sixty minutes. Carrying and swinging the hand weights helps keep your arm and hand bones strong. If you squeeze down on the weights, it helps your forearm bones as well.

Good daily exercise also includes the following: jogging (twenty to thirty minutes), jumping rope (twenty minutes), cycling (thirty to sixty minutes), and aerobic workouts (thirty minutes high impact, fifty minutes low impact). Swimming, although not a weight-bearing exercise, also is good if you do laps and maintain a brisk pace for thirty minutes or more. Romping around in the water will not work.

Bone is a complex matrix that includes collagen, a special protein that sort of holds things together. Collagen production calls for adequate dietary protein and vitamin C. However, because you have already recognized your need for vitamin C from the first three chapters, you'll do just fine.

DO I NEED ESTROGEN SUPPLEMENTS?

I'm from the school that says estrogen is necessary for average women once they are past or even almost past menopause. Doctors look for the risk factors for osteoporosis described on page 97 in deciding whether to prescribe estrogen.

Some articles suggest that estrogen increases your risk of cancer. It does very slightly, but like all things in life, it comes down to which risk is worst. By reviewing your genetic history of female cancer (breast and cervical), your doctor can tell if the risks are high enough to justify not taking the low levels of estrogen necessary to offset osteoporosis. For the vast majority of women, the real, large risk of osteoporosis is a far greater danger than the almost nonexistent risk of cancer from the hormone. In addition, the level of estrogen required can be minimized by the use of a second hormone, which reduces the extra cancer risk even more.

CHILDBIRTH

Although I am an advocate of not smoking during pregnancy, some women can't quit. Those women should take some calcium precautions to protect themselves and their child. Chapter 10 focuses on protecting the newborn baby; here I'll focus on the mother's bones.

Childbirth extracts an added burden on the mother's bone reserves because her body is called upon to produce a second skeleton. If Mom doesn't get enough calcium, nature takes it from her bones, which increases her risk of osteoporosis and the likelihood of a smaller-than-normal baby. There's an axiom: "Nature always favors the offspring unless the mother won't survive." Recent research also suggests that when dietary calcium doesn't meet this extra calcium demand, the shortfall causes high blood pressure, often seen in the later stages of pregnancy. This high blood pressure works against mother and infant, so don't let it happen to you.

There's only one solution to the pregnancy dilemma: Get more calcium. Strive for 2,000 milligrams daily. You can hardly get this much from your diet unless you use lots of dairy products. The most practical solution is a good calcium-magnesium supplement.

WILL ALL THAT CALCIUM CONSTIPATE ME?

Most people who start taking enough calcium incorrectly think they're becoming constipated. In fact, however, their stools are becoming more dense because about 60 percent of the calcium gets excreted. It makes for firm stools, especially if you take the multivitamin-mineral supplement that provides iron as well. Iron and calcium together produce firm stools.

However, remember our discussions of fiber? If women get at least the 30 grams of fiber they need daily, 77 percent of them will have no problem with constipation. The 23 percent who are naturally constipated should use the fiber-laxative supplements I described. As I mentioned, our bodies really can't get too much fiber.

A BONUS FROM SMOKING?

You might have been wondering, if smoking reduces my estrogen level and accelerates osteoporosis, what else happens? The answer is, you run a somewhat lower risk of breast cancer! Several studies have turned up a negative correlation between smoking and breast cancer. (A negative correlation means the smokers have a lower rate of breast cancer than nonsmokers.) That's good news.

So, if you take the advice given so far, you'll be reducing your elevated risk of several types of cancer, osteoporosis, and you'll have a lessened likelihood of getting breast cancer. While it isn't going to impress an insurance agent, it should help you gain peace of mind.

ADVICE TO MEN

Osteoporosis rarely affects men, for several reasons. Men consume more calcium and tend to satisfy their RDA for calcium longer than women, until they're into their twenties. In modern societies, men do more weight-bearing exercise longer into their adult life. And another plus for them is the fact that they don't bear children and don't experience menopause.

Consequently, men don't begin experiencing a decline in bone density until their mid-thirties or even their early forties. Because there's no menopause to accelerate the loss in bone mass, the decline is slow but it is steady. The longer men live, the greater their probability of osteoporosis—especially if they smoke, drink coffee, and eat meat.

Indeed, men now have a life expectancy into the mid-seventies, and many men will live to the ripe old age of one hundred. Not surprising, older men are showing up with osteoporosis. Though the numbers don't approach the statistics of women, it nonetheless foretells of a time, probably in the next century, when men will routinely have osteoporosis unless they take preventive steps.

The same rules that apply to women apply to men: Calcium and exercise are the keys to osteoporosis prevention. Indeed, there's no therapy, only prevention. Consequently, when I say that women who smoke should get 1,200 milligrams of calcium and daily exercise, the same advice is prudent for men.

PREGNANCY

S moking and pregnancy don't mix well. Children born to women who smoke are more likely to be smaller, and 60 percent are more likely to be born prematurely and develop respiratory problems, such as asthma, in their early years, and have behavioral problems. Worse yet, the children are more likely to have a cleft lip and palate. Because experts classify low birthweight as a birth defect and cleft palate is a defect, it's correct to say smoking causes birth defects. The goal of avoiding birth defects and premature delivery should give a prospective mother the strength to quit smoking before or, at least, while she's pregnant.

Being a realist, however, I know there are many women who cannot quit smoking while they are pregnant. Women who smoke or live with a smoker and plan to have a child should take the recommendations in this chapter very seriously and strive to exceed them in food and food supplements.

PRE-CONCEPTION NUTRITION

Not many years ago, if a woman thought she was pregnant, her doctor usually said: "Come and see me after you've missed two periods." That approach to pregnancy is as obsolete as yesterday's newspaper. Nowadays we know that pregnancy preparation should begin three months *before* conception. We call this pre-conception health and nutrition. Indeed, nutrition is preventive medicine and food is the vehicle of its practice. There is no better application of the concept of prevention than with pre-conception nutrition.

Birth control and our knowledge of conception has become so precise that most couples can plan the day of conception. Women should prepare their bodies to meet the challenges and demands they will experience during pregnancy. More important, by improving their own health status and building extra protective capacity against the effects of smoking, women give the baby a major chance at better health.

The objective of pre-conception nutrition is to build the mother's body so it will serve her and her child best during pregnancy. If the mother chooses to nurse her baby after birth, following the pre-conception nutrition plan can help make that period supportive to the baby and protect the mother's health as well. (See "To Nurse or Not to Nurse?" later in this chapter for reasons why I don't think it's good to smoke while nursing a baby.)

WHAT PRE-CONCEPTION NUTRITION ACCOMPLISHES

You have already begun by reading the previous chapter about preventing osteoporosis. You can take one of the most important steps toward successful pregnancy by getting between 1,500 and 2,000 milligrams of calcium daily and engaging in a sensible amount of weight-bearing exercise. This combination will build or, more likely, rebuild strong, dense bones. If you continue this calcium regimen and exercise appropriately while pregnant and nursing, you will retain this extra bone strength after the baby is born. So you'll improve your own health permanently.

Although it's not known with certainty why infants born to smoking women have a low birthweight, two pretty good theories were recently confirmed in research at the Harvard Medical School. First, smoking reduces the oxygen-carrying capacity of the blood. Hemoglobin, a protein in our red blood cells, imparts the red color to blood and carries oxygen to all our tissues. During pregnancy the mother's hemoglobin carries oxygen to the infant's blood system as well. Carbon monoxide from smoking, living with a smoker, or even from working in a smoky environment increases the amount of carbon monoxide in the blood. Carbon monoxide, a product of combustion, attaches to hemoglobin better than oxygen and blocks its oxygen-carrying ability. This reduces the blood's ability to carry oxygen and means that mother and baby don't get as much oxygen as they would if the mother didn't smoke. The solution is twofold: increase blood-borne antioxidants, which can trap carbon monoxide and spare hemoglobin, and build more hemoglobin as healthy red blood cells. In short, pregnant women should increase the total oxygen-carrying capacity of the blood.

A second theory teaches that nicotine causes tightening of blood vessels in the placenta. The placenta is the organ that develops in the womb so that nutrients can pass from the mother's blood into the infant's blood. It's an elaborate natural exchange center where the two circulatory systems come together but do not comingle with each other. This tightening of the blood vessels is not confined to the placenta only. It's also another reason that smoking causes high blood pressure in women, especially in the last three months of pregnancy.

Obviously you can't eliminate nicotine if you choose to smoke during pregnancy. However, by following the advice in Chapter 6, and using the omega-3 oils, you can help counter this nicotine-constrictive effect.

Other materials in smoke, the oxidants, destroy many nutrients. These include all the antioxidant nutrients, such as vitamins C and E, selenium, beta carotene, other carotenoids, and the special antioxidants in cruciferous vegetables. A large reservoir of these antioxidants is necessary so the baby can build its protective antioxidant reservoir. These antioxidants also neutralize the oxidants in blood, which helps its oxygen-carrying capacity.

Cleft lip and palate are variations of what are called neural tube defects. The neural tube develops during the first eight weeks of pregnancy. This tube, which will be the baby's backbone, can't develop correctly if sufficient folic acid isn't available. As mentioned, this B vitamin is likely to be short in average diets and especially in the diet of smokers. And, smoking can destroy folic acid. The shortfall plus the destruction of folic acid add up to trouble, and could explain why cleft palate and lip occur with high frequency in children born of smoking mothers. Consequently, we must pay special attention to the B vitamins, especially folic acid, in preconception nutrition and during pregnancy.

There's even something you can do to protect your baby against developing asthma. Although we don't understand asthma prevention, we can learn from people who live in areas where asthma is rare. Surprisingly, their diet is rich in the same omega-3 oils that will help reduce the constrictive effects of nicotine. So, if you've been following the advice in this book, you've already got a head start.

BUILDING RED BLOOD CELLS

Red blood cells are so important that several organs in the body are well equipped to build them. Indeed, in the time required to read this paragraph, your body, mostly in bone marrow tissue, will make about 100,000 new red blood cells. If you can boost that natural production of blood cells by just 1 to 3 percent, you'll have a dramatic head start on your planned pregnancy. In fact, some theories predict this should even reduce the likelihood of morning sickness.

During the first three months of pregnancy, your body will make an enormous amount of red blood cells to meet your increased need to carry oxygen to the baby. Hence, we know your body has the extra capacity to build these cells; it's just a matter of getting it started early.

Hemoglobin is an iron-containing protein. It follows that if your diet is rich in protein, you'll have a good supply of hemoglobin. But if you're a typical American woman and not using an iron supplement, you are getting about 12 milligrams of iron daily, which is 30 percent short of the 18 milligrams you need. If you are using the multivitamin-multimineral supplement I recommended earlier, you'll be getting about 30 milligrams of iron. This is more than enough for normal red blood cell production, but our objective here is a little higher.

To build hemoglobin-rich red blood cells, you've got to convince your body that you need more oxygen-carrying capacity and give it the tools to build that capacity. Therefore, you need to supply the iron needed to make hemoglobin as well as a few extra nutrients and to start an aerobic exercise program. I'll discuss the supplement first.

You can simply double up on the multivitamin tablet or capsule that I recommended. However, it would be better to take an iron supplement daily. A good iron supplement also contains some vitamin C, which improves iron absorption. By doubling your multivitamin or taking an additional 15 milligrams of an iron supplement, you will build your daily total to about 45 milligrams.

Using iron supplements along with calcium can increase stool hardness and make them difficult to move. In fact, you might feel constipated once you start this program. Fiber and lots of water are the best combination to counter hard stools and constipation. Purchase a fiber supplement, described in Chapter 5 (be sure it's made only with fiber and contains no laxative), and use it daily. Eat a high-fiber cereal daily and follow the diet plan in Chapter 17.

Exercise and correct fiber act synergistically on bowel regularity. Eat plenty of fiber-rich foods, exercise in the morning, and chances are that you'll begin to have a regular bowel movement every morning before you start exercising. This regularity will improve many body functions as well as skin tone. Exercise is one of the best means of helping all body functions become consistent.

Aerobic exercise is discussed in more detail in Chapter 12. Before you start this program, read Chapter 12 and determine your maximum heart rate. Also be sure you're free of any illnesses that would prevent you from a good exercise program. Since you're planning to become pregnant, you should definitely be healthy enough to exercise before pregnancy. After you're pregnant, consult with your doctor before beginning any exercise program. Here I'll give you the bare bones so you'll see what you need to accomplish.

Aerobic exercise is exercise where air is required. This means exercising so you breathe hard or are just on the verge of running out of breath. That rules out brisk walking and easy swimming. Indeed, it calls for jogging, rapid cycling (stationary bikes are fine), jumping rope, swimming, and exercise devices, such as a cross-country ski simulator, stair-climbing simulator, or a rowing machine, to name a few.

Your objective is to increase your pulse rate to about 80 percent of capacity, say to between 135 to 150 beats per minute, and keep it at that level for fifteen minutes. Do this at least five days each week.

Start slow. You might not be able to jog or jump rope for twenty minutes at first, so jog for two minutes, walk and catch your breath for one minutes and slowly increase the jog times until you can do the entire twenty minutes. Your body will get the message and will slowly put its hemoglobin-building capacity into gear.

BLOCK NICOTINE'S CONSTRICTIVE EFFECTS

Nicotine is thought to constrict the blood vessels in the placenta. This slows the passage of nutrients from the mother's blood to the infant's blood supply, and thus limits the child's accessibility to them. This constriction is like cutting back on nutrients, sort of a minor starvation, that produces low birthweight in the child and limits the level of oxygen going to each organ. Can a pregnant woman who smokes do something to relax the blood vessels and counter this constrictive effect?

There is no clear and direct answer to this question. However, we do know that substances called prostaglandins control constriction and relaxation of blood vessels. Your body produces these hormonelike substances from oils you get in food. The objective is to give your body the prostaglandin building blocks.

Your diet probably has an abundance of the omega-6 oils, such as corn oil and other widely used vegetable oils. The omega-6 oils produce the prostaglandins that tighten blood vessels. If you're typical, your diet is probably short in the omega-3 oils that the body needs to make the blood vessel—relaxing prostaglandin. You can change this balance by eating fish, using oils rich in the omega-3 oils, and using omega-3 oil supplements.

By starting three months before pregnancy, you will actually be able to alter the fat distribution in your body enough to make a difference when you become pregnant. Continue through pregnancy and, by the third month, or six months after you start your program, you will have achieved a good level of the omega-3 oils.

The body needs about six months to shift its content of the omega-3 oils enough to make a difference. This knowledge has been derived from clinical studies on people who have inflammatory diseases. Although these people start feeling results in a month, careful measurements have proven that it takes about six months to achieve the full effect.

How do you get enough omega-3 oil? That's the bottom-line question, and there are several approaches.

One way is to learn to eat the omega-3-rich fish described in Chapter 6. Four or five servings weekly is excellent; it's truly a case of more is better. You might be concerned about the observation that fish sometimes contains minor levels of toxins, such as lead, mercury, and pesticides. Many articles are written to create public concern for justifiable reasons, but, on average, ocean fish are safe. An alternative is to select hatchery-grown trout and salmon which are carefully regulated.

Flaxseed oil is an easy way to take omega-3 oils. A tablespoon added to your high-fiber cereal is a very convenient way of getting the best balance of omega-3 oils. Flaxseed oil can be purchased in most large health-food stores. It is amber in color, tasteless, and should be kept refrigerated. You really can't take too much of this oil because your body converts it to the active omega-3 oils as you need them. Some recent research reported from Tufts Medical School suggests that one of the oils in flaxseed oil, alpha linoleic acid, is especially important.

Omega-3 oil supplements are often sold in capsules as marine-lipid supplements. These capsules usually contain all three omega-3 oils; generally you'll need to take three capsules to get about 1 gram of omega-3 oils. Check to see how many capsules are required for about 900 to 1,100 milligrams of omega-3. Use this measure to decide which product is the better buy.

PREVENTING ASTHMA IN YOUR BABY

Although clinical support is thin, there's plenty of reason to expect the omega-3 oils will help prevent asthma in your baby. In areas of the world where women eat a diet rich in omega-3 oils, asthma is rare. Add to that the observation that many people in these areas smoke, including some expectant mothers, and you have some circumstantial evidence that says: "It can't hurt and might do a lot of good."

There's a surprising amount of information that suggests the omega-3 oils are therapeutic for asthma. In fact, people have used flaxseed oil since the time of Hippocrates—since about 450 B.C.

Finally, continue with the supplements while nursing your baby and you will have plenty of the nutrients essential to developing brain and eye tissue. You see, fish really is brain food, because that's one human tissue where these oils are absolutely essential. It won't hurt to give your baby a head start and improve your own health in the process.

I'm frequently asked how a nutrient a woman takes can affect the health of her baby. Besides the bad evidence from toxins, such as alcohol and nicotine, circumstantial data have emerged that a number of children's illnesses are related to the mother's diet. These include a form of childhood arthritis, a form of heart disease called cardiomyopathy, and even childhood brain tumors.

BLOCK THE TOXIC EFFECTS OF SMOKING

Antioxidants are as important for the developing baby as they are for the mother. However, it's tougher for the baby to get them from the mother's blood. In order for antioxidants to transfer to the infant's blood supply, the mother must have a higher than normal supply in her own blood. This is necessary because of how nutrients and toxins go from the mother to the infant.

The placenta consists of myriad small blood vessels from

the mother's body and myriad vessels from the infant. Though they don't allow blood to flow from one body to the other, they allow nutrients and toxins to pass from these small capillaries of the mother across the space between them, which is mostly fluid, and into the infant's blood. Similarly, but in reverse, toxins from metabolism in the infant's blood move into the mother's blood and are removed by her kidneys.

This exchange of nutrients and toxins between mother and infant works very well. Indeed, it works so well that even the smoke toxins easily pass into the baby's blood. However, they don't pass back quite as easily because of a simple physical property of fluids that are separated by membranes, as in the placenta.

Biological membranes, such as in the placenta, allow the nutrients and toxins to pass from regions of high concentrations to regions of low concentration. Because the mother does the smoking, it follows that her blood will have a higher concentration of oxidants and other by-products of smoke, including nicotine, than the baby's blood. So the toxins pass easily to the baby. Because of its immature liver, the baby's body cannot destroy the toxins. However, we can take advantage of the placental transfer system with the antioxidants and build the baby's reserve.

It's understandable that if the mother keeps a high blood reservoir of known antioxidants, such as beta carotene, vitamin C, vitamin E, and selenium, the baby will get a higher level from the placenta transfer. Moreover, if the mother eats a diet rich in cruciferous vegetables, the baby will obtain these antioxidants as well. Although we don't know to what extent the baby can build higher levels of its own protector substances, a better diet plus supplements in the mother gives the baby the best chance. Therefore, I recommend the antioxidant levels listed on Table 10.1.

Although the supplement recommendations may seem high, they aren't according to some experts who would recommend more. Consult the section "What Will Your Doctor Say?" if he or she objects to this plan. You also might balk at the extra servings of cruciferous vegetables, red vegetables, and fruit. However, these amounts of vegetables will help

TABLE 10.1
DAILY ANTIOXIDANT PROTECTION
FOR PRE-CONCEPTION AND PREGNANCY

	Pre-conception	Pregnancy
Vitamin C	1,000 to 2,000 mg	2,000 mg
Vitamin E	400 to 800 IU	800 IU
Selenium	150 mcg*	150 to 300 mcg
Beta carotene	25 mg	35 mg
Cruciferous vegetables	*Minimum* of two servings daily from pre-conception through nursing.	
Tomatoes and red vegetables	Minimum of one serving daily from pre-conception through nursing.	

*Mcg stands for micrograms, a unit of measure equal to one one-thousandth of a milligram.

you and the baby. If they are eaten steamed, raw, or with a minimum amount of dressings, the calories they supply are negligible. Therefore, all you must do is find those you like and eat them regularly.

TAKE EXTRA B COMPLEX

In Chapter 4 I discussed the B vitamins and explained how a smoker's basal metabolism is higher than average. The human need for B vitamins is directly proportional to the rate of metabolism. In this chapter I've recommended that you start an exercise program which will increase your metabolism even more. These factors, combined with our objective of building more red blood cells to expand your oxygen-carrying capacity, add up to a need for more B vitamins.

If you've wondered why I don't recommend extra folic acid, it's because you need to get all the B vitamins. Once you're pregnant, your doctor might prescribe a prenatal capsule that has extra folic acid. However, it's still correct to take all the B vitamins together.

Follow the recommendations in Chapter 4 and take a B vitamin supplement if you aren't already taking one. Your supplement should follow the guidelines I established earlier. These extra B vitamins serve your needs very well.

WATER

As I've mentioned, your body calls for about 64 ounces of water daily. Most of us aren't likely to drink that much water directly, but we get it from the beverages we drink, such as coffee, tea, and soft drinks, and even from vegetables and fruit. Remember, vegetables and fruit are about 75 to 80 percent water by weight.

Pregnancy imposes special demands on your excretory system. Your body must process the extra by-products that come from the infant and from the added processes your body must develop. Indeed, while your kidneys process about 50 gallons of blood daily when you're not pregnant, they must process about 60 to 70 gallons during pregnancy.

Water is absolutely essential for the kidneys to remove toxins from the blood and pass them out in the urine. More, water also is essential so your stools will be easily moved and sufficiently hydrated. Well-hydrated stools are about 75 percent water, which means they are especially good at removing toxins.

All this adds up to at least eight full glasses of water daily. You should drink one glass at each meal, one when you take your supplements, and one with each tablespoon of fiber. These seven or eight glasses are essential, so don't compromise.

COFFEE

Although you might not be able to stop smoking during pregnancy, I urge you to drop coffee. Excess coffee consumption is not good during pregnancy. For example, caffeine enters the infant's blood, but the infant's liver can't metabolize caffeine rapidly enough to clear it from the blood, so it remains there for longer than it should.

No studies have evaluated the combined effects of coffee and nicotine on fetuses. However, since both caffeine and nicotine are handled by the liver together we can speculate that the combination demands more of the liver than either one alone. Therefore, if you've chosen to continue smoking, I strongly recommend eliminating coffee. In any case, the consumption of plain water will help your body clear both caffeine and nicotine.

TO NURSE OR NOT TO NURSE?

Generally I'm in favor of nursing a newborn baby. Mother's milk is a unique formula that contains all the nutrients and protector substances a baby needs to thrive. Moreover, the composition of mother's milk changes as the baby grows to meet its changing nutritional needs.

However, environmental toxins find their way into mother's milk. It follows that if a nursing mother smokes, the baby is getting some nicotine and other chemicals in smoke. That can't be good for the baby.

Indeed, more and more experts are counseling pregnant mothers not to nurse their babies if they continue to smoke. Because I'm not an expert on this subject, I'll counsel caution. And because I think nursing is better, follow or exceed the pre-conception nutrition plan faithfully if you continue to smoke. Also speak with the baby's pediatrician about the issue of smoking while you nurse.

WHAT WILL YOUR DOCTOR SAY ABOUT THIS PROGRAM?

Your doctor will give you similar advice: Stop smoking (and other tobacco use) during pregnancy. I sincerely hope you will follow that recommendation. However, if you choose to continue smoking, you should discuss the steps I have suggested. In the next few sections I cover questions your doctor might raise.

Suppose the Doctor Questions High Levels of Vitamin C

Many years ago it was proposed that vitamin C at levels of 1,000 or more milligrams during pregnancy could cause what was tentatively called rebound scurvy. This hypothesis was based on two babies, born of mothers taking lots of vitamin C, with mild gum sores. According to this theory, during pregnancy the developing infant becomes accustomed to high blood levels of vitamin C. After birth, the baby's blood levels drop to normal, and, so the hypothesis taught, the infant's body reacted as if it were deficient. You might think of it as a relative deficiency of vitamin C. Subsequent research has proven that this type of rebound scurvy does not occur.

My objective in building high vitamin C levels is to neutralize some of the chemicals, mostly oxidants, in tobacco. When vitamin C neutralizes these chemicals, the effective level of vitamin C is dramatically reduced. Because the tobacco chemicals are transferred across the placenta to the baby's blood, it is essential to continue with high levels of vitamin C throughout pregnancy.

Suppose Your Doctor Questions Other Antioxidants

Vitamin E and beta carotene have been tested for safety at over 3,000 IU of vitamin E daily and 300 milligrams of beta carotene daily. That's beyond any level you'd be likely to use. (I've covered both nutrients and selenium in the book entitled *Prescription for Longevity*. Show that book, which has an extensive reading list, to your doctor if he or she expresses any doubt.) These antioxidants can do much good and no harm.

Suppose the Doctor Questions Omega-3 Oils

Omega-3 oils at high levels—about 16 or more grams daily—cause some changes in blood-clotting tendencies that could be risky for some people who are at high risk of stroke and heart attack. You aren't using an extra 16 grams of omega-3 oils. You're using a level that's similar to eating an extra daily serving of salmon.

So, ask your doctor if it's okay to eat an extra 3.5 ounces of salmon. If he or she says no, and you're not allergic to salmon, you'd better consider another physician. My aim is for you to counter the effects of smoking on your health and your baby's.

ONE LAST PLEA

After reading this chapter you might have a renewed interest in stopping smoking during pregnancy. Do it. Stop! But go ahead with the plans I've outlined for pre-conception and pregnancy. Because the residual effects of smoking last for about a year, these steps will help counter them, and you'll be healthier for keeping to the program. Your baby will benefit even more than you.

CHAPTER ELEVEN

INFANTS AND CHILDREN: NOT FOR PARENTS ONLY

About fifty ailments in children are linked to the passive smoke they breathe from parents. Recently, Dr. Anne Charlton of Manchester University in England published a review of 143 scientific studies, spanning twenty years, concerning how children are affected by passive smoke.

Most conditions aggravated by passive smoke are minor. They include sore throats, irritated eyes, sneezing, and coughing. However, some are very serious, such as crib death, meningitis, cystic fibrosis, pneumonia, asthma, some forms of heart disease, and higher risk of cancer later in life. Some of these conditions, such as cystic fibrosis, are congenital and, while not caused by passive smoking, are made significantly worse. Many of these ailments, such as meningitis and pneumonia, are caused by exposure to germs. However, children exposed to passive smoke are more susceptible to these illnesses and smoke aggravates them. Dr. Charlton's recent finding that more crib deaths occur in smoking households is surprising. Because the basic cause of crib death is unknown, it's probably a case where smoke aggravates the causative conditions. My objective here is to discuss what you can do, as a parent, to reduce the risk of any of these illnesses.

A best approach is to either smoke outdoors or set aside a "smoking room" where your infants and children aren't allowed. This suggestion will reduce dramatically, but not eliminate, their exposure to smoke. You can take other positive approaches to protect your children from the effects of passive smoking: Start them eating the right kind of diet and taking food supplements.

No one knows the extra nutrient and antioxidant needs of children who breathe passive smoke. It's safe to say their needs are significantly greater than the average; in my opinion, possibly two or three times greater, if not more. And it's important also to recognize that these children will not get these levels of nutrients from their diet if they're average and live in an average home. Therefore, supplements are absolutely essential, but let's start with diet first.

Chapters 17 and 18 outline the Smoker's Longevity Diet and illustrate it with a week of menus. This plan also applies to children who live with passive smoke. Their food intake will be adjusted by the amounts they eat, so don't try and foist adult servings on them. Rather, let them eat the amount they are comfortable with. Simply don't offer "junk food" alternatives, and most likely they'll eat the food that's good for them. I've never seen children starve when offered wholesome food, even if the parents have to "wait them out." Children will learn to like good food if they see their parents setting a good example. Most children aim to please, so give them a correct but realistic target to aim at. Don't worry if they put a little butter or even sugar on vegetables. It may look "gross" to you, but the object is to get them to eat.

Supplements are another matter. Once infants are off formula and on foods, doctors usually prescribe incomplete, horribly sweet supplements in liquid form. If you look carefully in drug and health-food stores, you can usually find a supplement that supplies all seventeen nutrients listed on Table 11.1 in a powdered form that needs to be mixed in milk or juice. Powdered supplements mixed this way work well for infants through about age two or three. Just don't save the unused portion more than about one day in the refrigerator. Toddlers from about age two and a half up until they're about four or five can take a complete, chewable supplement. Most children's supplements are highly flavored, but if you search you can usually find one that has a moderate flavoring and isn't sweetened to a fault. If they take two or three times the normal, single tablet, don't worry. It's perfectly safe.

TABLE 11.1
NUTRIENT NEEDS FOR CHILDREN
1–3 AND 4–6 YEARS

Nutrient	Ages			
Vitamins	**1–3**		**4–6**	
Vitamin A	400	R.E.[1]	500	R.E.
Vitamin D	400	I.U.[2]	400	I.U.
Vitamin E	6	I.U.	7	I.U.
Vitamin C	40	mg	45	mg
Thiamin, Vitamin B_1	0.7	mg	0.9	mg
Riboflavin, B_2	0.8	mg	1.1	mg
Niacin	9	mg	12	mg
Vitamin B_6	1.0	mg	1.1	mg
Folic acid	50	mcg	75	mcg
Vitamin B_{12}	0.7	mcg	1.0	mcg
Minerals				
Calcium	800	mg	800	mg
Phosphorus	800	mg	800	mg
Magnesium	80	mg	120	mg
Iron	10	mg	10	mg
Zinc	10	mg	10	mg
Iodine	70	mcg	90	mcg
Selenium	20	mcg	20	mcg

[1]R.E. = Retinol equivalents; 2,250 micrograms beta carotene or 5,000 micrograms of carotenoids.
[2]I.U. = International Units

Once a child is five or six years of age he or she can generally swallow a complete supplement. At that age extra vitamin E and C, and beta carotene supplements are also appropriate. These extra supplements will build an ongoing antioxidant reservoir that gives the child an added measure of protection. Another step is to mix a teaspoon of flaxseed oil in their food, such as cereal.

Fiber is as important for children as it is for adults.

Getting children to take fiber is quite easy, because they seem to like breakfast cereal and fruit. Select a cereal that has at least 4 grams of fiber per serving. A child's serving, topped with some fruit, provides essential nutrients and gets a child off to a good "fiber start" in the morning. Follow the advice on fiber in Chapter 5 and give your child a fiber supplement. Just use about one-third to one-fourth the adult serving size. Mix it with real fruit juice and you've added some extra nutrients to the child's diet. It all helps to meet the elevated need of children of smokers.

Additional protection against a smoky environment is derived from active play outside in fresh air. Read Chapter 12 on exercise and think children, instead of adults, and similar activity with less time. Children are naturally active, so the best thing to do is to get them to enjoy being active outdoors. This exercise has the same benefits for them that it does for adults. Make sure they are outside regularly, and keep active.

Children are natural snackers, so use this natural tendency to advantage. Encourage them to snack on fruits, such as apples, pears, oranges, and grapes, and easily eaten vegetables, such as carrot sticks and celery. Fresh fruit and vegetable juice supply the same nutrients. There is no way they can get too much of these healthful foods, and every bit they eat helps protect them a little more from the chemicals in the smoke they're exposed to. Be wise: Encourage a healthful diet, exercise, and proper supplements to help your children overcome the ill effects of passive smoking. It's the future you're protecting.

CHAPTER TWELVE

EXERCISE FOR SMOKERS

Most smokers I talk to are convinced smoking is so bad for them that it's a waste of time to exercise. "Exercise is like sending good money after bad," a smoker friend said to me. Nothing is further from the truth. I believe the average smoker can benefit more from regular exercise than a nonsmoker. Exercise not only counters many bad effects of smoking, but it will improve the physical health of a smoker just like anyone else.

While exercising, the temperature inside your muscles increases to about 102 degrees from its normal 98.6 degrees Fahrenheit. That 3.4 degree rise (1 percent) increases the rate of metabolism over 17 percent, which increases circulation by at least 100 percent. This change in circulation brings more oxygen to all organs and tissues, including the brain, and, at the same time, flushes toxic wastes from your body. It's like a spring rain cleaning dirty streets. That's why regular exercise reduces the risk of cancer, heart disease, and just about every known disease.

In Chapter 4 you met the B-team of vitamins. Your need for these vitamins is determined by your size and energy use. Exercising and smoking both increase energy expenditure, so it follows that your body will rely more on the B vitamins to stay healthy. Follow the guidelines cited earlier so you will not fall short in these essential nutrients. They are necessary for good health.

For reasons not well understood, smokers have more

abdominal fat. This shows up as a slightly higher waist-to-hips ratio in men and women; smoking is not sexist. Although it seems minor, this ratio is a good index of heart disease. A careful study proved that smoking has the ability to increase the waist-to-hips ratio; this finding, along with the oxidant effects discussed in Chapters 2 and 3, explains why smokers have more heart disease.

However, every problem creates an opportunity. You can reduce your waist-to-hips ratio by exercising. Indeed, if you follow the programs in this chapter, you'll reverse this tendency within six to twelve months. It's one more reason why smokers can benefit more from exercise than average, non-smoking folks.

STAN'S STORY

Stan is an old friend, an astrophysicist by profession, and a smoker since before age eighteen. At age thirty-five Stan was so out of shape that he would hack, cough, wheeze, and burp whenever he had to climb a flight of stairs. His doctor, friends, and relatives told him to quit smoking. He didn't. I told him to start jogging. "But," he said, "I smoke. Jogging will kill me and won't do me any good."

"Hogwash," I said. "It won't kill you any sooner than anyone else who's out of shape. Smoking is no excuse for not exercising. It'll do more good for you than it will for a nonsmoker."

I challenged Stan to meet with me every morning when I jog. We didn't jog together at first because I was in shape and he wasn't. However, we'd meet after our jogs and Stan would have a smoke while we talked. About eight months after he started jogging, Stan could jog alongside me and do 2.5 miles at 7.5 minutes a mile. Yes, he still has a smoke after his daily jog, but in his own words, "I've never felt better in my life."

I can add that Stan has never looked better. His physical condition is good. His skin has gone from a dull "smoker's gray" to a bright, healthy olive. He also follows all the advice in this book. So, follow Stan's lead and gain a new outlook on life.

PHYSICAL EXERCISE IS IMPORTANT

Every organ and tissue in your body improves if correctly exercised. By exercising regularly at the right level, you gain and maintain lean body mass, increase heart output, and reduce blood pressure. Exercise will keep you from becoming fat and help build a reserve capacity necessary to reach your optimum potential in every aspect of life. It helps you mentally as well as physically.

Exercise increases muscle mass, improves muscle tone, and changes muscle chemistry for the better. Lean muscle has a higher basal metabolic rate (BMR) than untoned muscle, because its chemistry is different. By exercising, you increase muscle mass, thereby reducing total body fat and increasing your overall BMR.

The quality of all lean body mass is interrelated. Improving muscle tone is accompanied by better bone density, which means stronger bones and slower aging. You also are rewarded with a better posture and, if you are a woman, a lesser likelihood of osteoporosis, and the shattering bone fractures that can occur in old age for both men and women.

A HEALTHY HEART AND STRONG MIND

Moderate, regular exercise improves cardiac output, reduces blood pressure, and increases lean body mass. Many studies have shown that regular exercise (for six or more months) reduces blood pressure by about 9 percent. This is an average. A recent study reported in the *Journal of the American Medical Association* showed the blood pressure reduction for many people in the study amounted to 13 percent. On average, the reduction was about 9 percent. For some people, a 9 percent blood pressure reduction will remove them from the "high blood pressure" category and put them into the "high-normal" category. With a little dietary effort added to the exercise, they're "home free," as the saying goes. But I must repeat the old caveat: You've got to exercise regularly, and it takes time for the results to be obvious.

Improved cardiac output means the heart pumps more blood with each beat. In other words, regular exercise improves the pumping efficiency of the heart. Put another way, it builds your heart into a stronger muscle. You gain reserve capacity because you have more heart-output potential than you usually need.

Now that shouldn't surprise you; after all, the heart is a muscle, and how do you improve the strength and flexibility of any muscle? Exercise, that's how! So, regular moderate exercise will improve the muscles being used in the exercise, including the heart. But every study confirms that the exercise must be done regularly and steadily to have this effect. Regularly means at least five times weekly, and steadily means that the effects start to be obvious in about a month but are really clear in six months. After a year there's no comparison to the starting point.

Moderate means that the exercise has to be vigorous enough and last long enough each time to have an effect— you need to sweat a little—but not vigorous so you are constantly sore, tired, or exhausted. In fact, people who overdo exercise do themselves more harm than good. Good exercise translates to vigorous walking for about forty to fifty minutes daily or jogging twenty to thirty minutes. There are many other forms of exercise that work well or better, and we'll explore these alternatives.

UNEXPECTED BENEFITS

Exercise is synergistic. That means that its sum is greater than its parts. Simply put, if you add the benefits of exercise to your dietary program, you get something even greater than you would have imagined.

Satisfaction comes with accomplishment. We humans, like all other creatures, respond to positive reinforcement. You will begin to find mental satisfaction as you gain physical flexibility, shift fat to muscle, and can perform tasks you once had thought impossible. But that's no different from doing anything well. Mental alertness always improves with exercise, because improved muscle tone brings improved circulation. Improved circulation brings more oxygen and nourishment to your master organ, the brain. It's not surprising that people who exercise are more alert and mentally quick.

Sleep will be sounder, not because you are tired; on the contrary, you will have more energy. You sleep better because everything about your body is more efficient. And although the restorative power of sound sleep remains a scientific mystery, no one can ever doubt its miraculous value, both mental and physical.

Regularity of bowel function will improve, another of the synergistic benefits of exercise plus diet. Although dietary fiber improves regularity and bowel function, regular exercise tones all muscles, including those of the bowel, and helps the bowel to respond easily and regularly. People who exercise regularly have better intestinal tone and are less likely to get intestinal disorders, such as diverticulosis, irritable bowel syndrome, and hemorrhoids. A recent study shows that people who exercise have a colon cancer risk about half of those who don't exercise.

CAN YOU DO IT?

No one is so unfit, so overweight, so physically handicapped that he or she can't exercise. I have had the beautiful experience of seeing eighty-one-year-old women start an exercise program to help their arthritis. My own mother, at eighty-five years old, mounts a stationary bicycle regularly and pedals for ten to twenty minutes. I have run so many 10K races against wheelchair athletes, blind runners, runners with arms missing, and once with a man who had an artificial lower leg that I no longer accept a physical handicap as an excuse. If they can do it, so can you. There's an exercise available for everyone; similarly, there are excuses available to everyone. It's too bad that the two easiest forms of exercise are running from personal responsibility and jumping to conclusions.

"But, Dr. Scala, I don't have time." Bologna! Nothing is as important as your health, but nothing is so easily avoided or put off. You'll just have to get up earlier, change your eating pattern, or stop work earlier. You can find the time in the twenty-four hours of each day.

"It's dark and dangerous in the early morning or early evening!" No excuse! The plethora of excellent indoor exercise devices available nowadays that have been tested and proven effective make it possible never to go outside. I'll even name some of them for you.

I'll make a proposition. One of the benefits of regular exercise is that you'll require less sleep. So, if you get up earlier, it'll become habit and you'll never miss the time. Time can be found if you want it!

"But, Dr. Scala, I'm so out of shape and I've been smoking so long that it'll take too long for me to get in shape." Look, it doesn't take as long to get into shape as it took to get out of shape. Furthermore, you should start slowly and work up. Indeed, a good start is to walk thirty minutes at a vigorous pace each day. That doesn't even require special shoes—just ones that don't cause blisters. Work up to a fifty-minute walk and you're on your way.

WHAT KIND OF EXERCISE?

Aerobics are the most efficient exercises for improving and maintaining general body fitness. *Aerobic* means "air," but specifically, the oxygen in the air. Your muscles need oxygen to function, and their need for oxygen goes up dramatically when you exercise long enough. Steady exercise—at least twelve minutes for very active exercises, such as fast rope jumping; usually at least twenty minutes or longer for others, such as jogging, and forty minutes for brisk walking—will produce aerobic conditioning.

Regular aerobic exercise, correctly carried out, does more to tone and firm the muscles than any other type of exercise. It is the most efficient way to remove muscle fat and to increase muscle metabolism—and your muscles will not get fat again if you maintain the fitness program.

Pushing a muscle steadily for the correct time, by jogging or walking, leads quickly to loss of fat and to good toning. Stop-and-go exercises, such as tennis, don't accomplish the same thing as quickly. Nonaerobic exercises, such as weight lifting, take a long time to remove muscle fat. They don't condition your heart muscles. In fact, most strong weight lifters can't run a mile because the general condition of their heart and arteries is often poor. Weight lifting is called anaerobic exercise, which literally means "without air."

AEROBIC VERSUS ANAEROBIC EXERCISES

Aerobic means with air; anaerobic means without air. This is a slight misnomer because you do still breathe when you do anaerobic exercise, but you don't exercise your heart and arteries and elevate your general metabolism. By elevating general metabolism, as in jogging ten to twelve minutes or more, you build your entire cardiovascular system. That's why this type of exercise is called aerobic. Your heart and arteries, indeed, your entire cardiovascular system, is mostly muscle and requires exercise more than any other system in your body. By doing some form of aerobic exercise, you prevent the buildup of fatty deposits in your heart and arteries and even remove some. As mentioned earlier, these deposits are the foundations of heart disease; preventing or eliminating them through exercise is one of the most important ways you can prevent heart disease.

In contrast to anaerobic exercise, aerobic exercise works large muscle groups, such as the arms and legs, challenging the cardiovascular system. In this way, major muscle groups and the cardiovascular system are conditioned together. Aerobic fitness produces entire body fitness.

Obviously, aerobic and anaerobic are the two extremes of exercise. Aerobic exercise is steady exercise of long duration. Anaerobic exercise is exercise of short duration. Table 12.1 classifies different exercises by type.

Aerobic exercise will produce a training effect (see Table 12.2) for average people, if done long enough. To achieve this effect, you must run for a minimum of twelve minutes or walk briskly at least twenty minutes. These times are determined by how long it takes for your heart to reach a "training rate," which I will explain shortly.

Anaerobic exercise, such as running a 100-meter dash, causes your heart to beat very rapidly, because you have created an oxygen debt by using energy from reserves without air. You breathe rapidly because your heart and lungs are only trying to "catch up" to repay the energy debt you have created while those reserves are restored. Oxygen is required to restore the reserves, so we call it an oxygen debt. Weight lifting, for example, seldom causes your heart to beat very

TABLE 12.1
EXERCISES CLASSIFIED
BY AEROBIC CONTENT

Aerobic (Long duration)	Stop and Go (Intermediate)	Anaerobic (Short duration)
Cross-country skiing	Badminton	Croquet
Cycling	Calisthenics	Field events
Jogging	Downhill ski	Golf
Jumping rope	Football	Isometrics
Rowing	Handball	Lawn bowling
Running	Racquetball	Sprinting
Stationary cycling	Tennis	Weight lifting
Trampoline-rebounder	Volleyball	
Walking (brisk)		

rapidly unless you create an oxygen debt, as you can do in the sprint, and it is simply catching up again. You can convert an anaerobic exercise into an aerobic one. A good example would be lifting a light weight rapidly up and down for about twenty minutes or more. But it is much better to jog, jump rope, or swim, because these exercises are far more effective and involve many muscle groups, not just one.

Tennis is stop and go. Unless you are very unusual, you have got to play tennis for at least two hours to get a training effect. If an amateur tennis player gets a high heart rate, it is usually due to an oxygen debt and not a training effect. Golf, in contrast, is a good way to ruin a healthy walk. You walk, stop, swing, talk, then walk some more. Your heart never gets to a moderately high, steady beat to establish a training effect.

A TRAINING EFFECT

"Training effect" is scientific jargon for saying that you have done something that has exercised and improved your cardiovascular system. You probably also have helped to build muscles, such as those in your legs and arms, in the process.

When you finish, you are in better condition than when you started. Seems worth doing, doesn't it?

To get a training effect, you are required to:
- Achieve a training heart rate (next section) quickly and do the exercise for at least twelve minutes, preferably twenty minutes. **Or**
- Achieve an increased heart rate and keep it up for at least thirty minutes and preferably one hour. **Or**
- Combine the above two requirements by achieving a modest increased heart rate and keeping it up for at least twenty minutes and preferably forty minutes.

You also should do the exercise on five out of seven days. Exercise is effective only when it is done regularly and with some rest periods, such as a day off every three or four days. Once you have been exercising one way regularly for a year and are in shape, it is a good idea to use several forms of aerobic exercise on different days, or weeks, to improve. You will improve because each exercise has its own benefits.

TRAINING HEART RATE

For most people, a training heart rate is about 80 percent of their maximum heart rate. (Maximum is the fastest rate at which your heart can beat.) Some well-trained athletes will achieve the maximum during exercise under the guidance of an expert coach. But most world-class athletes train at 85 percent of maximum. So, most experts conclude, if average folks get up to 75 or 80 percent of maximum, they are getting an excellent, safe training effect.

Table 11.2 lists maximum heart rates and 75 percent of maximum to guide you. The last column lists the 10-second pulse rate you should aim for, so you can keep track of your progress. Multiply this 10-second rate by 6 to get your heart rate per minute. Once you get into a regular exercise program, you will need to take your pulse only occasionally to make certain you are not overdoing or underdoing your exercise. I have been doing aerobic exercises for years and I don't bother taking my pulse anymore.

TABLE 12.2
TRAINING HEART RATES
(FOR AVERAGE PEOPLE)

Age	Maximum	75% Maximum	10-Second Pulse
20	200	150	25
25	195	146	24
30	190	143	24
35	186	140	23
40	182	140	23
45	179	134	22
50	175	131	22
55	171	128	21
60	160	120	20
Over 65	150	113	19

WHAT IF YOU CAN'T
ACHIEVE 75 PERCENT MAXIMUM?

Don't worry! Some people have a lower, resting heart rate. At age fifty-seven, my resting heart rate is 54 or less; the average for my age is 72. I don't achieve 128 very easily, so I don't bother trying. I get a good training effect at about 90 percent of the average for most people. If your heart rate is low, you are already blessed with a good cardiovascular system; strive for about 90 percent of the training rates given in the table. For me, that's about 115 to 120. You can figure yours out from the chart.

However, there is one rule for folks like us who don't get to a training rate easily. We need to exercise longer in each session! The price for better-than-average health is to work a little harder to keep the gift you have and do even more work to make it better. Look at it this way: You received a precious gift that is worth preserving. While working harder can mean running or walking faster, doing it longer is better; then you don't place as much wear and tear on your joints.

WHY EXERCISE REGULARLY?

Regular exercise builds and tones the cardiovascular system, including collateral circulation, which is the development of small arteries in the muscles in and around the heart. These extra blood vessels improve your health and aerobic capacity. When you exercise regularly, new blood capillaries start developing. It is as if your body decides you are into exercise for keeps and wants to open new avenues of nourishment for your tissues, so your body starts developing new channels to get oxygen-laden blood to the increased muscle mass. When you exercise regularly, you will notice that a difficult exercise becomes easy all at once. You have been making slow progress and suddenly real progress comes in one leap. That is because the new blood channels take time to make, but they open all at once. Think of it as a big, road construction project where all the new roads open at one time. It is like that with your body; suddenly you can do things you thought you would never achieve, because you have opened new muscles.

Your brain works the same way. As a student, did you try hard to learn something seemingly impossible, perhaps a process in math? Then one day it was easy, like a revelation. It is the same with exercise. Only in your brain, new neuron networks open all at once, and they give you a new thought pattern. Ponder this for a moment and you will realize that you can condition your mind to succeed, just as you can condition your muscles.

WHY EXERCISE DOES MORE FOR SMOKERS

Smoking puts carbon monoxide into your bloodstream. Carbon monoxide reduces the oxygen-carrying capacity of the blood by tying up hemoglobin, the protein that carries oxygen. In fact, a two-pack-a-day smoker loses about 7 percent of oxygen-carrying capacity, and a three-pack smoker loses 10 percent or more to carbon monoxide. It's almost that bad for people who work in poor environments. Smokers must increase their oxygen-carrying capacity by about 10 percent to stay even with nonsmokers.

Seen from another vantage point, by smoking you have reduced your physical aerobic capacity by at least 10 percent and more. I say "more," because you're also taxing your lungs' ability by forcing them to deal with smoke. If you build a higher capacity than average, you can cancel out these effects and build your aerobic capacity beyond its normal levels.

You're doing what athletes accomplish by training at elevated altitudes. At altitudes of say 5,000 feet, the air pressure is lower than at sea level, and the cardiovascular system must work harder to obtain sufficient oxygen. When athletes train at that altitude, their bodies respond by building more capacity than normal. Then, when they compete at lower altitudes, they have a better-than-average cardiovascular capacity and their athletic performance isn't limited by their oxygen-carrying capacity. As a smoker, you're doing the same thing by exercising regularly. Your blood will respond by building its capacity. However, your brain is skeptical and you must prove you're in it for keeps. Once convinced, your brain will instruct the system to go ahead and build.

OXYGEN DEBT

All exercise requires oxygen. The same, basic combustion process that lets the engine of your car burn gasoline is at work in your body. Both require oxygen and fuel: gasoline for the car; glucose and fat for your body. However, unlike your car engine, your body can exercise without oxygen for brief periods. But when it goes without oxygen, you have got to pay back the oxygen debt without delay. That's why when we climb the stairs fast or when we swim underwater for short distances, we are out of breath.

A short burst of activity, such as running for a bus or climbing stairs, leaves you gasping for air and your heart beating quickly. This happens because your body used high-energy materials to let you perform and didn't burn your glucose all the way to carbon dioxide. It let you create an oxygen debt.

To pay the oxygen debt, your heart beats quickly and you breathe fast to get blood to your lungs. When your blood passes through your lungs, you get rid of the carbon dioxide and take on more oxygen. Your liver and muscles then use the oxygen to process the wastes they have built up, and you pass the carbon dioxide to the air on the next pass of the blood through the lungs. No man-made engine can duplicate this process we carry out every day with such ease. If you stop the air to your car, it will simply stop running.

However, creating an oxygen debt doesn't build a good cardiovascular system. It doesn't even build a reasonable reserve for future situations, so don't even consider using it for training; it will not work.

But you can build yourself up for short-term, aerobic exercise. Did you ever notice that sprinters run long distances to build capacity? Then they use short-distance sprints to build their muscles and timing for the sprint. But their capacity comes from aerobic training. They build their anaerobic technique onto an aerobic foundation; doing so correctly requires an expert coach.

THE BEST AEROBIC EXERCISE FOR YOU

Different strokes for different folks, as the saying goes. The best aerobic exercise for you is the one that you will do regularly, consistently, and long enough to achieve a training effect. Then you will keep it up for the rest of your life. Look over Table 12.3 with a view toward picking the exercises you like best. It lists three groups of aerobic exercise by the approximate time required to develop a good training effect. In each category I have listed the approximate time necessary to achieve a training heart rate and then the time for a conditioning effect. Less vigorous exercises require longer exercise time.

You can modify most of these exercises to meet your own needs. Let's go through each group from left to right and discuss its good and not-so-good qualities.

- Group 1 consists of exercises for people who are already in good condition. These are borderline anaerobic exercises that can be done long enough to get a training effect. If you haven't been exercising, you are likely to develop sore muscles from doing them. It is also difficult to exceed the twelve-minute minimum

TABLE 12.3
TYPICAL AEROBIC EXERCISES

Group 1 1–1.5 min. to THR* (12 min. minimum)	Group 2 3 min. to THR (30 min. good time)	Group 3 8 min. to THR (50 min. good time)
Bench step	Aerobic dancing	Bicycling
Jumping jacks	Cross-country skiing	Brisk walk
Jumping rope	Jogging	Skating
Running in place	Rebounder	Swimming
	Rowing	

*Training heart rate.

due to boredom and the pounding in one place. Exercises in the other two groups are easier.

- Group 2 exercises can be done by anyone who is reasonably healthy. Some exercises, such as jogging and aerobic dancing, can be done in organized groups. Others, such as cross-country skiing and rowing machines, involve the use of equipment. The rebounder or minitrampoline is a device that works well in a small room. Even jogging can be done on a machine in the home, office, or gymnasium.

- Group 3 exercises are the best starting group for everyone. Heart patients can find a place here and paraplegics can do wheelchair workouts. You can bicycle in the country or on a stationary exercise bicycle in your home. Either ice- or roller-skating works well. These exercises can be done in a group or solo. You just have to devote at least twenty minutes daily. I recommend you start with forty minutes and work up to an hour. Forty minutes seems like a long time, but that is what it takes to get your cardiovascular system working at the right level. It's not easy to regain health: no pain, no gain.

EXERCISE EQUIPMENT

Almost every aerobic, outdoor exercise can be duplicated in the home. You can even watch television while cycling, jogging, rowing, cross-country skiing, and climbing stairs, among other activities. Technology has made it possible for everyone to become physically fit without leaving the house. A few rules apply.

- Never use motorized devices. The motor is spending the energy, not you.
- You get what you pay for. Studies have shown that the most effective devices are more expensive.
- Simple is better. The best devices require you to use your arms and legs actively. You don't need added heart monitors and other electronic gadgets.

I am frequently asked which exercise device is best. There is no single answer. I rank them in the following order:

- Cross-country skiing machines. These devices exercise the arms and legs independently. You work all the major muscles and don't "pound" your joints.
- Stationary bicycles. These require you to use your arms and legs at the same time. They develop resistance by air resistance as the wheel turns. The only minor flaw is that the arm and leg exercise is linked together. Therefore, they are not quite as good as cross-country skiing, because one exercise powers the other and the total effort is divided between the two.
- Stationary joggers, treadmills, and stair-climbers. These are excellent for the legs and can simulate hills or be as difficult as you need it to be. The only drawback is that your arms are generally inactive; in fact, they are less active than if you actually jogged or climbed stairs.
- Rowing machines. These can be excellent if they have an independent arrangement for leg exercise with a movable seat. Most of them exercise the upper body very well; if they have a moving seat, the legs get good

exercise as well. If you have got leg trouble or have lost use of your legs, you can't beat these machines because you can do the upper body alone.

AEROBIC DANCING

Some people like to exercise in a group or under the guidance of a leader-instructor. Aerobic dancing, more commonly called "aerobics," is the thing for them. It requires an instructor-leader who sets the pace according to the fitness and physical limitations of the group. So, "aerobics" are available for the most physically fit, professional athlete, and for people with serious arthritis.

"Low-impact" aerobics are available for people with joint problems or who are seriously overweight. In contrast, when you are advanced enough, you can do aerobics wearing hand and foot weights to burn extra calories and strengthen muscles. In short, there's an aerobic-dancing level for everyone.

BASIC STRETCH AND TONE

Every aerobic exercise program should include about fifteen minutes of stretching and toning. These are exercises that require you to stretch the tendons in your arms and legs. They also should force you to exercise muscles in hard-to-reach places. They can be as simple as you want them or as elaborate as you need. You should always do a few basics. Do each one ten times at first, working up to thirty daily.

- Situps. With knees bent, situps—effective even if only done partway—help to strengthen and tone abdominal muscles. Put your arms behind your head and try to reach your knees with your elbows.
- Leg raises. Lying on your back, then on each side, raise one leg, hold it up for a second, and put it down. This tones muscles inside the thighs and helps reduce their fat. Helps get rid of cellulite!
- Hip rotation. These are done standing with legs spread. Touch each leg in turn with the opposite hand, and come straight up after each.
- Hip reduction. Stand straight, hold 10 to 20 pound

weights with your hands together waist high. Rotate all the way to one side; then to the center; and then to the other side. This helps reduce waist fat.

- Stretch. Stand straight, cross your legs, and touch your toes in one sweeping motion starting with your hands together high over your head. Then cross your legs the other way and repeat. This help helps stretch leg tendons and keep them from getting stiff.

Video Workouts

There's no substitute for having an expert instructor. Television can bring one into your home. If you own a videocassette player, you can purchase or rent tapes for aerobics and stretch and tone at any level of difficulty you desire. You also can take time to learn each exercise correctly and progress at your own, comfortable pace. It is like having your own, personal coach right in your own home.

Getting in Touch with Yourself

Whatever exercise is comfortable for you is a good one to start with. Get in touch with your body by taking your pulse while resting, while walking at a moderate pace, and at a brisk pace. Try taking your pulse during a slow jog or when cycling; stop briefly to take it. Your pulse should be below 100 beats per minute within ten minutes after working hard; it should slow to normal within about twenty minutes. An easy way to take your pulse while walking or jogging is to grasp your neck gently under your jawbone with your left hand so your thumb can feel the back of your jawbone. Press your thumb in slightly and you will feel your pulse.

Become familiar with your heart and how it works. Take a brisk walk, jog, a brisk cycle, or swim to get your heart rate up; then stop and see how long it takes to return to normal.

When to Start

This moment is the beginning of the rest of your life, so now is a good time to start. By the time you finish this paragraph you will have 100,000 new blood cells and about 14,000,000 other cells. They can use the extra air. If you haven't been exercising, start slowly; a brisk forty-minute walk is an excellent way to start. Then progress to brisk walking for five-minutes; then a one-minute jog followed by five minutes walking, and continue in this manner for up to forty minutes. A healthy person with no leg or heart problems can maintain a twelve to fifteen minutes per mile pace for forty minutes or about 2.5 to 3.0 miles. A practiced, brisk walker will do ten minutes per mile. You can do the same with a stationary bicycle or any other device.

Experiment with different forms of aerobic exercise to find one that suits you and your life-style. Don't join an aerobics group right away; try it out first. Some people find they need a group and others can't stand a group. If you are a jogger or walker and like a group, you will probably be able to find one nearby.

WHEN TO EXERCISE

Most exercise programs fail from poor timing. Modern lifestyles are so complicated that both discipline and experimentation are necessary to find what is best for you. Here is what some of my smoking students have done.

Nancy, a private secretary: "I get up at 5:30 A.M. and go to a 6:00 A.M. one-hour aerobic class. I need a group! Not only that, my schedule is so busy that if I don't get it out of the way in the early morning, I will have at least ten reasons for not doing it after work."

June, a Ph.D. research chemist: "I jog for thirty minutes at lunchtime; then I do exercises for fifteen minutes. I do it alone and don't speak to anyone. That way it is just me at my own pace."

Jim, a business executive: "I use a NordicTrack [a cross-country ski] device for a thirty-minute workout at 6:00 A.M.; I watch the morning news. Then I do fifteen minutes of exercises. It is the only time I have no excuses. When I'm traveling, I jog at the same time."

Carole, an editor: "I get home at 6:00 P.M. and go for a thirty-minute jog in the winter or bike ride in the summer. It clears my mind and removes all the tension of the day. When I'm finished, the tension's gone and I'm at peace with the world. Even my children like me better." As you can see: different strokes for different folks.

Is There a Best Time?

"Best time" is in the eye of the beholder. However, physiology gives the edge to the end of the day and sociology to the beginning of the day.

Exercise not only tones the body, it relieves stress and tones the mind. Stress for most people is usually highest at the end of the day, so exercise then helps the mind as much as the muscles. However, the difference is slight because early-morning exercise provides a different advantage.

Any time you exercise, your brain produces natural opiates called endorphins, which elevate your mood so you become more optimistic. While they help you feel better after the day is done, they also help you start the day with an optimistic outlook. So, while evening is biologically a little better for exercise to relieve stress, its edge isn't large.

Sociologists have learned that people who exercise in the morning are less likely to quit, because most people have control of the early-morning hours before the day's obligations take over. There is no reason not to exercise; all you have to do is rise earlier and get started. Most studies also have shown that morning exercise makes you more efficient during the day. The efficiency is partly from an optimistic outlook and partly from the mental strength that comes with discipline. If you are a typical person, the morning is best.

Will I Be Tired?

No! People who exercise gain more stamina. Stamina is staying power: the energy that lets you keep going after ten hours as you were after one hour. Every study has proven that people who exercise regularly increase their stamina by a large measure over people who don't exercise. Look at it this way: Exercise makes your body and mind more efficient. Your metabolism is higher, but your heart works less to maintain the system. Your blood sugar doesn't fluctuate, so your moods remain at an even level. It all adds up to being more effective.

A conditioned body also seems to create an optimistic outlook naturally. I think it is the natural endorphins at work and the confidence that comes from accomplishment. Studies have been carried out on professional race drivers, business executives, secretaries, athletes, and housewives with the same results: condition your body and you condition your mind.

You have to love yourself to love life and love others. You must respect yourself to respect life and your fellows. It all starts with your body. Treat it with love and respect and the rest becomes easy. People who do this have more confidence in themselves, and they radiate it to their fellow men and women.

Start now!

CHAPTER THIRTEEN

SKIN: ITS NATURE
AND COLOR

We can make our skin look healthy and beautiful from the outside with creams, oils, and other agents. However, what goes on inside our body, specifically the results of diet and life-style, has a more dramatic and lasting effect on our skin color and tone. Even if you smoke, eating the right food and choosing the correct life-style will help your skin be supple and have a healthy glow.

Skin is your body's largest organ. It's about 6 percent of body weight and covers a large area. For example, a 120-pound, 5-foot 5-inch woman has over 16 square feet of skin weighing over 7 pounds; a 6-foot 2-inch, 200-pound man has over 21 square feet of skin weighing over 14 pounds. The lungs and small intestines have larger surface areas but not the proportionate weight. I urge you to purchase a book on the skin and learn about this marvelous organ, as our space does not permit us to cover it here in much detail.

Like all organs and tissues, the skin is made up of countless cells arranged in two major layers. The epidermis, the outer layer of the skin consists of two layers: an outer layer of dead cells (the stratum corium) and a lower layer of live cells. Below the live layer of epidermis cells is the dermis. The dermis is a live, vital tissue filled with small blood vessels, sweat glands, nerves, and other microscopic organs essential to the maintenance of the skin. Skin cells in the epidermis reproduce every three to six weeks depending on body location, health, general nutrition, and heredity. These cells reproduce from the bottom, so each new cell pushes the old one upward. As the old cells progress upward, they move farther from the vital, life-giving nutrients, including oxygen, in the dermis, and they can't eliminate their wastes, so they die. This progression means the the outer layer of the epidermis consists of entirely dead, dehydrated, flattened cells. They are made mostly of protein, pigments, some oils, and carbohydrate, and they slough off when we wash and scrape our skin against clothing.

Surprisingly, hair follicles from which hairs grow are actually appendages of the epidermis that extend deep inside the dermis. By residing deep in the dermis, and even into the tissue below the dermis, hair follicles are well nourished by blood vessels. These hair follicles produce cells that die and become part of the hair shaft.

Sweat glands, which originate in the dermis, are connected to the surface by tiny openings called pores. A pore often has a hair growing out of it, and the opening serves two purposes: one is an opening for the hair; the other permits water to be released. Sweat glands go deep into the dermis where they produce water for excretion at the surface. When this surface water evaporates, it removes body heat that helps keep your body cool in the summer and when you're working or exercising.

Sebaceous glands are often associated with the hair follicle. These glands produce oils that give the hair its sheen and make the dry epidermal cells more soft and supple. These oils also help protect our skin from the sun, dry air, harsh chemicals, and other environmental effects.

The network of blood capillaries in the dermis supplies the most important nutrient, oxygen, and removes the most important waste, carbon dioxide. These capillaries also transport everything that gets into your blood. If you smoke, they transport nicotine and some pigments from smoke. Consequently, sensitive people can smell the smoke in your skin, just as they can smell garlic on your breath.

SKIN RESPONSIBILITIES

Skin shields you from the sun, chemicals, bacteria, and countless environmental factors. It's waterproof so you don't swell up when caught in the rain or dry out when in the hot sun. At the base of the dermis, a layer of fat serves as a shock absorber to protect your internal organs, insulate them from the cold, and keep in body heat.

A marvelous network of nerves in the dermis, connected to the hair follicles, can simultaneously detect the slightest touch, temperature change, air flow, and even changes in barometric pressure. These same nerves sense environmental changes inside and outside your body. Your body then adjusts blood flow to either conserve or dissipate heat. So, when it needs to dissipate heat, the capillaries let blood flow to the skin, the sweat glands go into action producing water for evaporation, and heat is given off. Conversely, when it's cold out or you need to conserve body heat, the capillaries tighten and the skin doesn't get as much blood. Because the insulating fat layer is below the dermis, this marvelous system works independently to control body heat.

Changes in our hormones profoundly effect the skin; so do drugs and food. Therefore, caffeine, nicotine, alcohol, and our emotions cause changes in our skin. In this way our skin reflects our mood and lets those around us know if we're tense, stressed, relaxed, or simply feeling good.

NATURAL SKIN PIGMENT AND HAIR-EYE COLOR COORDINATION

We need vitamin D to survive and just the correct amount to thrive. Our bodies need vitamin D to absorb calcium from food or from calcium supplements. Cholesterol produced in our liver is carried by the blood to the dermis of the skin, where sunlight converts it to vitamin D. This vitamin D, after further changes in other organs, is responsible for intestinal absorption of calcium.

Too much vitamin D is toxic. It causes the body to deposit calcium in soft tissues, including major blood vessels where plaque is found, and in the kidneys. Rarely does a person produce too much vitamin D because the skin has several ways of filtering excessive, high-energy rays from the sun.

People native to equatorial areas between the Tropics of Cancer and Capricorn have thick, dark, sometimes black skin to prevent the sun's rays from penetrating it. In contrast, people native to the North, such as Scotland or Lapland, tend to have thin, light skin so it will trap the weak sun rays in those regions. People native to the temperate zones in between those extremes have the ability to produce pigment that filters sunlight. These people tan if exposed gradually to sunlight, as would happen in the natural progression from winter to summer. This ability to tan regulates the manufacture of vitamin D. In contrast, people from the North generally don't tan easily. So, if they're overexposed to the sun, they quickly become red with a burn. A burn prompts them to leave the sun and also filters the sunlight. A burn isn't the best way of avoiding excessive vitamin D, but it works.

Skin pigment and thickness evolved from humans' survival needs. Along with the need to modulate sunlight, there developed a general tendency toward thickness, dryness, and oiliness. These tendencies are no longer important, because we can spend our lives indoors, we have sunblocks, and we can get vitamin D in milk, dairy products, and vitamin tablets. But inherited factors make skin different.

In general, dark skin tends to be oily and well hydrated. In contrast, very light skin tends to be nonoily and dry. Think about oiliness and dryness for a moment and you'll see it goes with pigment. Skin likely to experience lots of sunlight can benefit from a thin oily layer to keep moisture in. Oils also help to modulate sunlight. In contrast, light skin needs to be thin and allow sunlight to pass through to make vitamin D. Thus our ethnic origins have an effect on the number of sweat and sebaceous glands our skin has.

Well, this lesson in evolution tells us where we came from and gives insight into why Italians are dark, tan easily, have oily skin and dark eyes, in contrast to Scots who are light, don't tan easily, have dry skin and light eyes.

Skin and hair color are usually coordinated. Color coordination isn't why; human survival is. Blue eyes are more sensitive for the lower, northern light levels, and light hair is more easily seen in dark light. Consistent with light skin, light hair is thin, not dense, and contains little pigment. Dark skin and eyes go together because dark eyes are less sensitive to the harsh light of equatorial regions. Like dark skin, dark hair is more dense with pigment.

This brief introduction to skin color can help you understand why light skin, hair, and eyes are more sensitive to smoke and fumes than darker skin, hair, and eyes. Light skin is more sensitive because it is thinner and has less protective oil and pigments, so irritants can penetrate more easily. Moreover, it will help you see why the skin of light-complected people is more likely to darken from smoking. I'll start at the beginning and work toward a plan for protection.

SMOKING AND SKIN COLOR

People often say that smokers have gray skin and thin hair. Some even claim smoking darkens their hair. All these observations are correct and are consistent with skin pigment, tobacco tars, and the effects of nicotine on the skin. Light-skinned people are affected most by smoking and dark-skinned people the least. Let's explore them one at a time.

Feed people enough carrots, carrot juice, or beta carotene capsules, and they'll turn orange. They turn this color because beta carotene accumulates in epidermal cells. Indeed, some enterprising people decided to make a profit from beta carotene's ability to color skin from within by selling capsules of canthaxanthine, a yellowish carotenoid pigment. Once in the skin cells, canthaxanthine imparts a tanned color. The federal government stopped the sales of canthaxanthine capsules because its sale was not within the food guidelines, which means a material must be generally recognized as safe.

Let's consider how skin color can change from excessive carotenoid ingestion. Carotenoid pigments move from the capillaries in the dermis to the epidermal cells. This transfer has a definite health advantage, because these pigments modulate sunlight and help protect skin, especially light skin, from the sun's harsh rays. In fact, enough beta carotene will help prevent a burn and produce a good tan.

Dr. Michaelin Mathews-Roth, a professor of medicine at

Harvard Medical School, used this fact to help sick people. She gave people with a severe, light-sensitive skin disorder enough beta carotene to color them orange. This level of beta carotene caused the skin to modulate light enough so these people could tolerate sunlight. While earlier people with this disease literally had to live in darkness, now they could be exposed to sunlight. Some of them could actually develop a tan.

All epidermal cells finally become part of the stratum corium and slough off. So people who ingest a lot of beta carotene not only take on an orange glow, but this glow will come off to some extent and impart a slight tinge to white garments. This fact proves that skin accumulates pigment and passes it off. Once more, Dr. Mathews-Roth proved large amounts of beta carotene are safe.

Pigments in tobacco that are carried in tobacco smoke have similarities to beta carotene, canthaxanthine, and other plant pigments. After these pigments are breathed into the lungs, some pass into the blood. For people who chew tobacco, the pigments pass into the blood through the digestive system. Once the pigments enter the blood, natural processes take over, and eventually they will find their way into the epidermis. If you smoke enough, one reason your skin will appear gray is because it's burdened with dark pigments found in tobacco smoke.

A second reason your skin appears gray is because nicotine causes the capillaries of the epidermis to become constricted. Constricted capillaries do not supply the dermis and epidermis with as many nutrients, especially oxygen. The result is the absence of a healthy glow, because the cells are being deprived of the natural pigments in blood.

STRATEGY FOR BETTER SKIN COLOR

You will return a healthy glow to your skin by restoring better nutrition and by supplying the correct plant pigment and lots of oxygen to build a healthy dermis and epidermis. This means following the advice for getting antioxidants, the diet strategy in Chapter 17, and the exercise program in Chapter 12. Let's review what each step accomplishes.

In Chapter 17 you will be introduced to a diet rich in

protein, low in fat, and correct in carbohydrates. A supplement plan to supply more beta carotene is also provided. Follow this plan and you'll get a variety of carotenoid pigments, including beta carotene, canthaxanthine, lycopene, and many others. In addition, you'll get all types of dietary fiber. This will keep you regular, but it also helps to eliminate tobacco pigments from your body.

By taking supplemental beta carotene, you will supply your skin with pigments that impart a pleasing glow. If you are a heavy smoker or have light skin, take more beta carotene for added protection and better skin color. It will take three to six weeks for the plan to start showing results, so a little patience is required.

Exercise will improve your circulation. Exercise increases metabolism, moves more blood to the body surface, and gets more oxygen to the viable cells in the epidermis. This increased metabolism speeds skin turnover and eliminates dead cells more rapidly. There is no substitute for exercise!

Exercise and B vitamins go together, as I discussed. Exercise and the B vitamins improve metabolism in the skin, increase circulation, the manufacture of cell components and the incorporation of carotenoid pigments into the dermal cells.

SKIN AND HAIR CONDITIONS

Smoking is hardest on light skin because it shows the color better, is thinner, and is less hydrated. Omega-3 oils and vitamin E can help. Both these nutrients will increase the surface oils by adding oils to the epidermis via the dermis and the sebaceous glands. Additionally, vitamin E keeps the omega-3 oils from being damaged by the oxidizing materials in tobacco smoke. If you've got light, dry skin, and you smoke, you're likely to have thin, listless hair. Hair is produced by a group of specialized epidermal cells in an appendage of the epidermis, which goes down into the dermis, where it is bathed with blood and the nutrients it contains.

So, by supplementing your diet and exercising, you improve the internal quality of each hair. It's a natural outcome of better nutrition. However, there's a little more you can do to add a nice sheen and give luster to each hair: Supplement your diet with omega-3 oils.

Each hair follicle has a small gland alongside of it called a sebaceous gland. As each hair grows outward, it becomes coated with the oil produced by the sebaceous gland. This coating creates luster and sheen to the hair. Adding omega-3 oils, vitamin E, and beta carotene to your supplement program increases the output of your sebaceous glands. The result is not only more supple, good-looking skin, but better hair quality as well.

WHEN DO I SEE RESULTS?

Improving skin is a slow process. Remember I said that skin cells reproduce every three to six weeks and sometimes longer. Therefore, if you start a program today, your skin won't be fully turned over for as much as six to ten weeks. That means you need to keep your program going for four weeks before people will start to notice. If you've been smoking a long time, it will take you longer to improve your skin because you've got more pigments to cycle out. So, perseverance is required, but it will definitely pay large dividends.

Better hair calls for even more patience. Hair grows about one-third of an inch to one inch a month. Consequently, if you start today and have average hair growth, you won't notice the results for about three months. Anything that develops as slowly as hair growth isn't usually noticed unless we make an effort. However, trust me; the results are worth it. If you want to see the results, take pictures every two weeks for a year; you'll be pleasantly surprised.

WILL PROTEIN HELP?

Most people, smokers included, get plenty of protein. However, if you want to make an added effort, a little extra protein will improve skin and hair growth. You can add protein to your diet with a protein supplement. Or, you can add an extra egg to your daily diet. Because you'll be eating more fiber and using a fiber supplement, the added cholesterol won't hurt. In addition, the oils and pigments in the egg yolk will improve the color and sheen of your hair.

PUTTING IT TOGETHER AGAIN

Table 13.1 sums up the steps you can take to improve skin and hair.

TABLE 13.1
SKIN AND HAIR IMPROVEMENT

- Antioxidant supplements: beta carotene, vitamin E and selenium, vitamin C.
- Stress-fighter vitamins: B vitamins, including all the B vitamins, with at least 100 percent of the U.S. RDA.
- Omega-3 oils: 1 gram daily (usually three capsules).
- Optional protein supplement; take about 15 grams daily. Or eat an egg daily.
- Diet: follow the Smoker's Longevity Diet in Chapter 17.
- Exercise: five days weekly for at least twenty minutes at a training heart rate.

You've probably noticed by now that many of the preventive measures I've described are somewhat repetitious. For example, you take antioxidants to prevent heart disease, cancer, cataracts, and emphysema. The omega-3 oils help prevent heart attack and stroke. Moreover, exercise helps all of these and even improves skin and hair color.

These improvements happen because the same nutrients and antioxidants have beneficial effects on all tissues. By focusing on skin and hair, I've chosen ones you're most likely to notice. In the next chapter we'll look at skin wrinkles and gum health.

CHAPTER FOURTEEN

SKIN WRINKLES AND POOR GUMS

For years dermatologists have said that people who smoke have more wrinkles than nonsmokers. In fact, this anecdotal observation has been recently confirmed by scientific research. It leads to a question: How can something you do with your lungs create more skin wrinkles?

Some dermatologists say it's because smokers must squint more, thanks to the irritation of smoke on the eyes, and squinting produces wrinkles if you do it long enough. To support their idea, they quote research that says the wrinkles are more prevalent around the eyes and on the forehead. It's a variation on the idea that if you do something strange with your face it will stay that way.

Biochemists, in contrast, look at the protein matrix that holds skin together. They say this protein, called collagen, is damaged indirectly by materials in smoke. In short, it can't be rebuilt correctly and so wrinkles develop in those places.

Both notions are correct. Nevertheless, the biochemist is probably "more correct" than the observer who says "It simply stays that way." By learning more about what happens to the collagen in forming a wrinkle, we can develop an approach to slow down wrinkle development.

NATURE'S NYLON

Collagen is often called "nature's nylon." It is a protein that forms a matrix of fibers throughout the dermis and the fatty tissue, or subcutaneous fat, just below the dermis. Like nylon, collagen is a fiber that is woven into a netlike matrix that has multidirectional strength.

From experience, you know that your skin can be pulled, twisted, folded, even compressed and still return to normal. Nylon also returns to normal when it's similarly tortured.

However, nylon is a homogeneous man-made fiber that looks the same everywhere; collagen is not. Collagen, like all proteins, consists of about twenty-two building units called amino acids. These twenty-two units are linked together into fibers, and small fibers are intertwined with each other until a large fiber is built. Then large fibers intertwine, and so on.

Collagen, like everything in the body, is in a state of dynamic equilibrium. That means it is being broken down and rebuilt anew constantly. Like skin, which is replenished, on average, about every three weeks when we're young and six to eight weeks as we get older, collagen is renewed regularly. And when any protein is remade, something can go wrong. That's why both notions about wrinkles are correct. But first we'll consider what can go wrong from the biochemistry of how collagen is made.

For the body to build collagen, or any other protein, it needs energy, basic materials, and vitamins and minerals. In general, the energy is available in the form of blood sugar. Basic materials are available if you eat a reasonably good diet; that's one place where smokers can improve. But several critical nutrients, including vitamin C and some B vitamins needed to make collagen, are destroyed by smoking.

In the last chapters I've discussed how oxygen, the king of all nutrients, can be a little lacking in smoker's blood. In addition, skin is a peripheral tissue (external), and smoking tends to cause peripheral tissue capillaries to tighten. Thus there are two reasons smokers might not have enough oxygen, an essential nutrient in energy production. In previous chapters an exercise and iron-supplement program was recommended to make up for that shortfall.

Once you've got the energy and the amino-acid building blocks, you need several vitamins, including vitamin C, some B vitamins, and the minerals zinc and magnesium. You've seen several reasons why these nutrients are likely to be short in supply in smokers. Smokers' diets are often short in vitamins and minerals to begin with. And smoking destroys vitamin C and some B vitamins. In addition, it imposes a greater need for the other antioxidant nutrients.

You know that getting plenty of antioxidants is the most efficient way to make up for this dietary shortfall and antioxidant destruction. Take at least 500 milligrams of vitamin C daily and up to 2,000 milligrams for insurance. Take beta carotene, vitamin E, and balanced B-complex supplements daily. The diet in Chapter 17 will provide the needed minerals, as will using a balanced vitamin-mineral food supplement and the calcium-magnesium supplement described in Chapter 9.

SQUINTING DOES AFFECT THE SKIN

You might wonder: If collagen is constantly being removed and replaced, why do wrinkles develop in the first place? That's where the "squinting" hypothesis is correct. Let's see what happens.

When you squint a wrinkle develops. In the small area where the skin folds, the cells and tissue are squeezed. Though it's not the same as severely restricting blood from your leg, say, so that you get cramps and a tingling sensation, by squinting you do restrict blood flow and nutrients to the area where you squint. Collagen synthesis doesn't take place at that spot for an instant, or for however long you keep squinting.

Stop collagen synthesis for a moment and it doesn't matter. But do it regularly every day, many times a day, and it adds up. In fact, cell reproduction in the area declines and a wrinkle, or crease, develops.

A good comparison is the depressions, called "pockmarks," often left from adolescent acne. The difference is that acne causes a loss of collagen and death to cells in the area because of the localized infection that caused it in the first place. So the area is depressed because of missing tissue. Cosmetically, it can be corrected by a "spot" injection of collagen made from animal tissue. Later I'll discuss cosmetic options for correcting smoker's wrinkles.

Another way to prevent wrinkle development is to practice not squinting. Smoke in areas where the smoke is blown away, so you won't have to squint or frown as much. But rest, with your eyes closed, and exercise can accomplish even more.

Exercise brings oxygen and nutrients to the skin. Whenever you exercise you increase the blood flow to your skin by at least 100 percent. If you exercise actively enough, your skin temperature will increase by a couple of degrees. Although this increase doesn't seem like much, the rate of metabolism, the building and renewing of body tissue, including the skin, increases over 35 percent.

Besides, exercise stimulates your body's production of a group of natural steroids we call anabolic steroids. Anabolism is the building of new tissue. These anabolic steroids actually stimulate protein synthesis. It's why regular workouts increase muscle mass and strength. They also build healthy skin.

Therefore, when I said there are many reasons for smokers to exercise regularly, beauty and the prevention of wrinkles should get their rightful place. You've learned how exercise improves skin color. Now you see that it also improves skin tone along with muscle tone.

PREVENTING WRINKLES BETWEEN EXERCISE SESSIONS

In Chapters 6 and 7 I discussed how smoking elevates blood pressure by increasing the constriction of small capillaries. I also explored the need for omega-3 oils. You might have skipped those chapters because you're too young to worry about having strokes or heart attacks, but now you have a good reason to read them. They will help you look better.

Briefly, the omega-3 oils, specifically one called EPA, help relax the blood capillaries. Think of them as countering, to some extent, the action of nicotine on the blood vessels. By following the dietary program in Chapter 17 and taking about 1 gram (1,000 milligrams) of omega-3 oils daily, you'll be taking a giant step in wrinkle reduction.

GUMS AND TEETH

Just as it works on the skin, smoking works on gum tissue. Gum tissue is a marvel of collagen production and saliva production, all organized to anchor and protect the teeth.

Although we hear much talk about how teeth are anchored to bone, we seldom hear that specialized collagen fibers do the anchoring. And similar to skin, gum tissue is attached to the teeth by collagen fibers. Though gum tissue doesn't wrinkle, a more insidious process takes place.

If gum tissue isn't kept healthy and strong, bacteria can grow in the area where the teeth and gums meet. These bacteria slowly can destroy the collagen fibers that anchor teeth to gums and bone. We call this periodontal disease. "Peri" means "around" and "odontin" means "teeth," so it's a disease around the teeth.

Periodontal disease gives an early warning called gingivitis, which is characterized by bleeding gums. People with gingivitis usually notice their gums bleed when they brush their teeth or even if they eat crusty bread. Their gums also bleed easily if they bump their mouths. It's not something to dismiss from your mind because it doesn't hurt or seems to pass quickly.

Research at Tufts Medical School showed that over 60 percent of gingivitis cleared up when victims regularly took 600 milligrams of vitamin C. This should come as no surprise because we know that vitamin C is essential for effective collagen production. And the basic cause of gingivitis is unhealthy collagen.

Unfortunately, the Tuft's research didn't focus on smokers, who have a higher incidence of gingivitis due to smoking. The research proved that some people simply need more vitamin C to build healthy gums. We can extrapolate their findings to smokers because we know with certainty that smoking destroys vitamin C. It follows that smokers with gingivitis require more than the 600 milligrams of vitamin C. It simply means that smokers are a variation in the human population.

But knowing what we do about the effects of smoking

on nutrient delivery to all tissues and its ability to destroy vitamin C, we shouldn't be surprised that it affects gum tissue as well. The solution, more specifically, the prevention of gum disease, lies in all the measures we've taken to produce healthy skin.

Therefore, the exercise, dietary, and supplement plans will help create healthy gums right along with fewer wrinkles. In short, though smoking or chewing tobacco might stain your teeth, if you follow the recommended routine the likelihood of your getting gum disease will be markedly lessened.

An added point should be made about beta carotene and the other carotenoids. The evidence that they prevent the development of precancerous (dysplastic) cells in tobacco chewers is testimony to their ability to protect gum tissue in general. If you've been following the plans in this book, you'll be helping yourself to healthy skin and gums. This can't help but make you look better and feel better about yourself.

COLLAGEN INJECTIONS

Cosmetic surgery has blossomed in recent years. Though we usually think of people having wrinkles erased and noses reconstructed, the objective of cosmetic surgery is much more humane. It has let seriously deformed people gain a new lease on life. Some have been able to come out of darkened rooms into the light and find the same happiness many of us take for granted. The surgeon's ability to help these people has improved things for everyone, and collagen injections are one improvement.

Collagen can be injected into the area of a wrinkle or pockmark and fill the void that exists. Voilà! The wrinkle or pockmark disappears and the person's skin looks smooth and supple. Obviously, anyone who wants to partake of this procedure must go to a dermatologist.

Collagen injections work for about six to twelve months and then need to be renewed. Renewal is necessary because of collagen's state of dynamic equilibrium. Consequently, they are not a permanent solution. Prevention is still the best cure.

CHAPTER FIFTEEN

SMOKER'S SKIN AND EMPHYSEMA

In older people, smoking causes the skin to appear stiff and leathery—I call this smoker's skin. Even though smoker's skin is generally studied, it's an observation most dermatologists willingly make. Even though smoker's skin is often labeled gray or wrinkled skin, it's not quite the same as the wrinkles and color loss we all get as we age.

However, there's no doubt that smokers are likely to develop emphysema. Smoking is at the top list of risk factors for emphysema, and whatever is in second place is a far second, unless you breathe chemical fumes and smoke all day at work.

I describe emphysema as imagining your lungs becoming stiff like old leather, instead of being a soft, supple, flexible tissue that can expand and contract as you breathe. That's a pretty good, albeit exaggerated, description of lungs with emphysema.

People who have emphysema describe life as "living out a nightmare." Their feet seem unbelievably heavy and they can't seem to move. People with this disease can't get enough oxygen from the air to do things we all take for granted, even simply walking.

These people's lungs don't work as they should. They can't expand and contract to get air into the small sacs, the alveoli, and get the carbon dioxide out. Consequently, when emphysema is advanced, they must travel in a wheelchair with an oxygen tank. By not walking, the amount of air they need is reduced, and the oxygen makes their remaining lung capacity more effective.

When I tell people that leathery skin and emphysema are the same thing in different tissues, they act surprised. They shouldn't because both are the result of accelerated aging that comes from environmental toxins. I'll explain the phenomenon and you'll quickly see the preventive steps to take.

PREVENTING SMOKER'S SKIN AND EMPHYSEMA

Proteins are made of some twenty-two subunits we call amino acids. Think of a protein as a large string of beads that contains twenty-two different kinds arranged any way you want. You can guess that there's almost an infinite number of proteins, because your string can have ten beads, ten thousand, or even more.

Think of folding and twisting the beads to get even more variety, because you can make almost an endless structure in that way. Now think of doing it with other proteins, and you get an idea of the protein and tissue variety available in nature.

But there's a problem. Toxic chemicals we call aldehydes can react with the subunits (the beads), and link them together. That is called cross-linking. So now review your concept: You can cross-link within one protein; cross-link among two, three, or even more proteins. When all this cross-linking occurs you form a rigid structure that isn't as flexibile as each string of beads or even a whole bunch of beads. In fact, it's as if the beads were taped together every so often between, across, and within strands. You'd have a massive structure and, if it was taped often enough, it wouldn't be very flexible. Excessively cross-linked skin collagen is like this excessively taped up network of beads.

What we just envisioned for beads is what happens in leathery skin and, worse yet, in lungs that have emphysema. The proteins, mostly collagen, have become so cross-linked that the tissue flexibility is gone. The tissue becomes thick, rigid, and loses its ability to stretch and contract. This cross-linking is used in the plastic industry to convert soft plastics to stiff, hard plastic. That's not good for lungs and skin.

Another problem emerges because, in smokers, the glands that produce fluid don't work as well. This means the skin will be coarse, because the sebaceous glands are no longer secreting oils and lubricating the dead cells of the epidermis. In the lungs, the quantity of aveolar fluid declines. This means the lungs are even less flexible and can't extract oxygen from the air as well as they should.

STOP CROSS-LINKING

Obviously, the best way to stop cross-linking is to trap the aldehydes. The best way to trap aldehydes is to cause them to react with vitamin E, other tocopherols, beta carotene, and all the antioxidants we discussed in earlier chapters. Further, exercise more to help flush them from your body.

HOW MUCH?

At the risk of sounding repetitive, I'll review a good supplement plan for smokers to assure them of enough antioxidants. Just remember, this plan is in addition to the dietary plan discussed in Chapter 17.

- Vitamin C: minimum 500 milligrams daily; preferably 2,000 milligrams daily.
- Vitamin E: minimum 100 I.U. daily; preferably 400 I.U. daily.
- Beta carotene: minimum 25 milligrams daily; preferably 30 or more milligrams daily.
- Selenium: 75 to 150 micrograms daily.
- B complex: 100 to 450 times the RDA daily.
- Mixed cruciferous vegetables: at least a one-cup serving daily. No exceptions.

WHY DO PEOPLE SMOKE?

Tobacco smoke contains about 900 clearly identifiable chemical components. Several have hallucinogenic effects and some can produce an intoxication similar to alcohol. It's easy to envision natives in Central or South America burning tobacco, inhaling the smoke, and feeling pleasant from the experience. Once they identified the source of the experience, you can imagine how they would pick out tobacco leaves and burn them selectively.

The Mayas in Central America and Indians of North and South America smoked cigars made from tobacco. Shamans—ancient medicine men or priests—believed tobacco helped create a good relationship with the gods they worshipped. Consequently, they encouraged its use and helped foster the cultivation and curing of tobacco.

Archaeologists have discovered that tobacco was chewed, used to make beverages, and the dried dust was sniffed. Just as tea was and is used as a beverage, tobacco leaves were infused with water to make a beverage. Special bowls have been discovered from which this beverage was drunk. Tubes and pipes also were made for smoking; cigars and cigarettes were later inventions of partly European origin.

Among the Maya, tobacco was used so extensively that primitive syringes were developed to administer tobacco enemas. Administered in this way, components of tobacco, including nicotine and other materials, would be absorbed into the bloodstream rapidly. There's no doubt that a person could get "high" from tobacco used in these ingenious and dangerous ways.

Experts speculate that tobacco enemas and other direct introduction of tobacco extracts into the body probably caused some serious illness and even death. Nicotine is very toxic if sufficiently concentrated, so without modern methods of analysis, primitive people could easily produce a toxic overdose.

Learning to use tobacco safely couldn't have been an easy task and much illness and some deaths were probably part of the learning process. Nicotine has some deadly properties that are fast acting. If highly concentrated in its pure form, nicotine is highly toxic and an excellent insecticide. Indeed, a strong concentrated infusion will kill most insects. A single drop of pure nicotine placed on a rabbit's skin can kill the rabbit.

Scientists have developed an index of toxicity by seeing how much of a substance is required to kill rats and mice. The level necessary to kill 50 percent of the animals is called a substance's L-D 50, meaning lethal dose to 50 percent. Nicotine has an L-D 50 of 0.3 milligrams per kilogram if injected intravenously or 9.5 milligrams per kilogram if simply injected into a body cavity, such as the abdomen. In practical terms, to kill a person who weighs 154 pounds (70 kilograms), I would need to inject only 21 milligrams (.02 grams) of nicotine into a vein or 665 milligrams (about 0.7 grams) into the abdominal cavity. Now remember, a teaspoon of water is about 5 grams, so 0.7 grams isn't even a teaspoonful.

Tobacco grown for commercial purpose contains about 8 percent nicotine. You'd have to chew an awful lot of tobacco in order to get enough nicotine to be even mildly toxic. It's what nicotine does for us at lower levels that we're interested in.

A LESSON FROM PRIMATES

Give a group of monkeys some tobacco, and before long you'll find them chewing it. In fact, they soon learn to put it in their cheek, just like people who chew tobacco. With a little instruction, monkeys can learn to smoke quite easily. Though monkeys prefer to chew, smoking gets the nicotine deep into their lungs, where it's absorbed into the blood very efficiently. Unlike people who experimented with tobacco extracts, injections, and enemas, monkeys simply chew tobacco and smoke it if taught how. Hence, monkeys in the wild never had to face the toxic nature of tobacco extracts.

In some societies, including the Maya, children learned to eat tobacco flowers. These flowers contain about 5 percent of the total nicotine in the plant, which is enough to provide users with a mild but nontoxic high. About 64 percent of the tobacco plant's nicotine is found in the leaves, 13 percent in the roots, and another 18 percent in the stems. So, harvest the leaves, allow them to cure and dry, and you've got most of the active ingredient. Tobacco curing is the slow drying and aging of tobacco leaves in a structure that allows air flow and shields the leaves from sunlight.

Curing tobacco leaves reduces the natural starches in them to sugars. This imparts a sweetness to the leaves that overrides the bitterness associated with the nicotine and other chemicals. Monkeys and baboons prefer cured leaves, and in the wild, they'll let them dry before using them. They learn to chew naturally. Many of them have learned to get juice out of pipes that researchers left behind.

Primates have learned to use other helpful plants in the wild, including some that have antibiotic properties, emetics, vermifuges to get rid of intestinal parasites, and others. Therefore, the fact that primates naturally learned to use tobacco confirms that tobacco has desirable properties, even if it is addictive.

Indians learned to cure tobacco, then mix it with sugar, anise oil, and other sweet resins. Primates learned to do the same things, and even have been seen mixing tobacco with sweet plant materials, including anise.

By observing how the primate's use of tobacco parallels human use, we can conclude that tobacco is desirable. In general, the leaf must be cured to reduce its bitterness. Once cured, it is enjoyed more mixed with sweeteners and tasteful resins, such as anise. Now we're ready to ask: Why do we use tobacco at all?

WHY WE USE TOBACCO

Much animal research has been conducted to try to understand what benefits tobacco use offers. Animals have been given nicotine under a variety of conditions, and their reactions mimic human reactions. Consider the following reasons people have given for their use of tobacco.

• "I can concentrate better when I'm smoking."

Animals that are given tobacco or nicotine and are taught to run a maze or perform a task do much better than animals not given tobacco. In addition to learning more quickly, the "nicotined" animals are more alert and more attentive.

These animal studies confirm what people say: that smoking helps in studying and learning. Indeed, many people, professors included, will tell you that they can't study unless they have a pack of cigarettes handy.

• "I can cope with stress if I'm able to smoke."

In a study of rats, a tone was heard before a shock was administered. By acting quickly, an instant after the tone was heard, a rat could press a lever and avoid the shock. However, the rats would freeze when the tone sounded and became rigid in anticipation of the shock. But rats given nicotine could overcome the stress that followed the tone, press the lever, and stop the shock. Even if the shock started, they would still press the lever. In short, the nicotine helped them deal with a stressful situation and control their environment.

• "Smoking calms me down. I feel relaxed and able to accept things."

Confine a large number of animals, such as rodents, dogs, or monkeys in a limited space and they become aggressive. In fact, in these studies observers tally the number of bites and aggressive acts. Give these same confined animals nicotine, and aggressive behavior declines greatly. Thus many animal studies confirm the human claim that tobacco has a calming effect.

• "Smoking lifts my spirits. I feel more cheerful."

No animal study can duplicate human depression, so we must rely on people's comments. Because most people confirm that nicotine, more realistically tobacco use, lifts their spirits, a clinical study was conducted on withdrawal. In a double-blind study, smokers were given an antidepressant drug, Prozac, to see if it would help them quit. The rate of successful quitting leaped from 16 percent to 64 percent. The only problem is that the smokers needed to stick with the Prozac.

This finding seems to confirm the fact that smoking helps depressed personalities. Put another way, nicotine might just be one of nature's most readily available mood elevators, or antidepressants, if you prefer to see it as a cure.

All this tells us that nicotine at nontoxic levels has many good qualities. It's a stimulant that helps people become more alert. But unlike some stimulants, it seems to improve concentration and make learning come a little faster. Nicotine also helps people cope with the world by calming their nerves and helping them deal with environmentally induced stress. And finally, it's a pick-me-up for people who tend to be a little depressed.

Is It Addictive?

We know that nicotine is addictive because, from a practical point of view, it's very difficult for people to quit smoking. Symptoms associated with withdrawal of other addictive drugs have been identified in people trying to quit smoking. These symptoms include tension, restlessness, irritability, increased hunger, an inability to concentrate, and insomnia. All of them can be relieved by giving these people more nicotine. So, indirectly, the process of withdrawal confirms that the active component in tobacco is nicotine.

Confirmation that nicotine is addictive comes from studying primates that were addicted to tobacco. They exhibit identical withdrawal symptoms. Hence not only humans are subject to nicotine addiction. It can happen to primates as well.

A FUTURE POLICY

Nicotine is not the only addictive drug in widespread use. Many, possibly most, adults become addicted to caffeine. Coffee, tea, and caffeinated soft drinks are accepted worldwide as beverages with a variety of social uses as well as for a "kick start" in the morning. However, in contrast to smoking, health-care professionals have not identified any serious illness-causing side effects to caffeine use.

In contrast, smoking's major side effects—heart disease, stroke, and cancer—result not from nicotine itself, but from other components in smoke and tobacco juice from chewing or snuff dipping. High blood pressure, however, can stem directly from nicotine. On the other hand, coffee oils are probably as toxic as materials in smoke. However, the coffee user gets only a small amount, because these oils must go through the digestive process, in contrast to smoking, which pulls the toxins directly into the lungs and facilitates their movement into the bloodstream.

Recently nicotine has become available in a gum and as a time-release patch similar to seasick medication. Though they are used now to help smokers quit the smoking habit, it's possible that this type of nicotine will take its place as a socially accepted drug like caffeine and alcohol. After all, both caffeine and alcohol are similarly toxic—in fact, deadly at high doses—and are just as addictive as nicotine.

Indeed, purified nicotine safely administered in prescribed patches provides the benefits of nicotine without the dangers of smoking or chewing tobacco. Compared to excessive coffee and alcohol use, it is completely benign. Do nicotine patches pose a dilemma for drug regulation?

An argument in favor of nicotine can be built on its ability to relieve depression, elevate the spirit, improve alertness, and facilitate learning. In a society that readily uses drugs to make people more manageable, nicotine seems quite benign. Caffeinated soft drinks represent a significant precedent for the addition of the physiologically active and addictive drug caffeine to widely used beverages by people of all ages. After all, if the purpose of a Coke or Pepsi is to quench the thirst, what's the caffeine doing there? Isn't it just possible that addicting kids to the caffeine in soft drinks is a way of ensuring future sales? Does the addition of caffeine to a soft drink pose a dilemma for drug enforcement? Or is it because we don't generally think of caffeine as an addictive drug?

CHAPTER SEVENTEEN

SMOKER'S LONGEVITY DIET

The Smoker's Longevity Diet puts the protector substances in food into everyday practice. It's a balanced diet by all the accepted criteria for good health.

Follow this diet, use the supplements I described, and I promise that, within a week, you will feel better than you have for a long while. You'll sleep more soundly at night and get up with more bounce in the morning. Within a month you'll look better and people will notice. Stick with the diet plan and your risks of cancer and heart diseases will decline in proportion to the length of time you follow the diet.

Other minor and, depending on your point of view, possibly more important benefits will accrue. Your skin won't wrinkle as quickly. You'll recover from minor ailments faster. You'll have more energy and be more alert mentally. If you're overweight, you'll drop the extra pounds. Add exercise, and you'll convert body fat to muscle. You'll be pleased with the "new you."

THE BEST HABIT YOU'LL EVER DEVELOP!

Many people live to eat. I want you to learn to eat to live. The Smoker's Longevity Diet is endless in variety—no two meals or snacks have to be the same. Once you work this diet plan into your life-style, it becomes habit. The best habit you'll ever develop!

THE SMOKER'S LONGEVITY DIET: PROTECTIVE EATING

Fruits and Vegetables: 7 Servings Daily

Determine serving size by comparing with the following examples.

VEGETABLES: ½ cup cooked or 1 cup raw
Examples: 1 large stalk broccoli with the floret; 6 medium asparagus spears; 2 potatoes without skin or 1 baked potato with skin; 1 medium raw carrot.

FRUIT: 1 medium apple, orange, pear, etc; 3 small plums or apricots; ⅛ large cantaloupe; ½ small melon; 1-inch slice watermelon.

Five Rules Apply

- Eat one serving of a cruciferous vegetable daily.
- Eat one serving of deep green or dark red vegetables, such as spinach, broccoli, sweet red pepper, carrots daily.
- Eat one serving of fruit raw, such as an orange, apple, or banana, daily.
- Eat three servings of beans, such as lima, red kidney, lentils, weekly. Change varieties regularly.
- Eat one serving of a mixed salad with tomatoes and onions daily.

Grains and Cereals: 4 Servings Daily

Determine serving size by comparing with the following examples.

CEREALS: ⅓ cup cold or cooked; use cereals that provide 4 or more grams of fiber per serving.

BREADS: 1 slice whole-grain bread or 1 whole-grain roll.

PASTA: 1 cup cooked (2 ounces dry).

GRAINS: ½ cup cooked.

- Eat one daily serving of a high-fiber, natural cereal with low-fat or nonfat milk. Try to eat three varieties of high-fiber cereals weekly.

Natural Bulbs: I Serving Daily

Serving size is variable. The following objectives apply: Eat garlic, onions, leeks, shallots, and chives regularly.

Examples: Use 1 clove of garlic to flavor a salad, soup, meat, spaghetti sauce, etc.; ¼ onion in your salad or with some vegetables; ¼ cup chopped raw leeks. Flavor foods with these bulbs regularly. You can't eat too many bulbs.

Milk and Diary Products: 3 Low-fat Servings Daily

Determine serving size by comparing with the following examples.

MILK: One cup (8 ounces)

YOGURT: 6 ounces

CHEESE: About 1½ ounces

- Although ice cream is a dairy product, one full pint is needed to fulfill the nutritional need. Frozen yogurt is somewhat better, because it contains fewer calories, but it still calls for 1 pint. Newer low-fat ice creams are better yet.

Protein-rich Foods: 2 Servings Daily

Determine serving size by comparing with the following examples.

FISH, FOWL (WHITE MEAT): 3½ ounces (about ¼ pound)

EGGS: 2 medium

CHEESE: 1½ ounces

BEANS: 1 cup cooked

Weekly Rules to Follow

- Eat fish at least four times; finfish at least three times.
- Eat one vegetarian meal; for example, pasta with cheese; eggs; beans.
- Eat fowl, such as chicken, turkey, or duck, as often as desired; remove the skin after cooking.
- Eat red meat only once weekly; never is better.
- Don't eat processed meats, such as bologna, hot dogs, and the like.

- Eat visible eggs (e.g., scrambled, sunnyside up) a maximum of two eggs three times weekly.

Oils and Fats

The best oils for:
FRYING: are peanut oil or butter.
BAKING: are canola or rapeseed oil.
SALADS: are olive, canola, walnut, avocado, and linseed.
- Add 1 teaspoon flaxseed oil to salad dressing and in baking to increase your intake of the omega-3 oils.

Water

- Drink four 8-ounce glasses daily. Use purified water, mineral water, or distilled water.
- Seek out water that is free of nitrates, chlorides, and man-made chemicals, such as pesticides. Water rich in natural minerals, including calcium and magnesium, is best.

For alternate food selections, the following source book is recommended: **Bowes and Church's Food Values of Portions Commonly Used**, 15th ed., revised by Jean A. T. Pennington.

I encourage you to go beyond the diet and include more fish, white meat from fowl, less or no red meat, and more vegetables and fruit than the advised seven servings. Become a fish-eating vegetarian and you'll accelerate the benefits of the diet and will live a better, healthier, longer life.

CAN YOU IMPROVE ON THE SMOKER'S LONGEVITY DIET?

Think of your body as a castle and the Smoker's Longevity Diet as its foundation. Although scientists will argue over megadosing on vitamins and minerals, there's unanimous agreement on the benefits of applying the principles of the diet with a heavy hand. A few easy additions will pay extra dividends. For example:

- Nine servings of fruits and vegetables daily is better than the basic seven.
- Fish six times weekly is better than four; and no red meat is better than any red meat.
- Extra cruciferous vegetables and foods from the garlic family will add to the benefits. Truly more is better.
- A high-fiber bran cereal daily is an excellent start for every day. Oat, wheat, rice, or corn bran are excellent for variety.
- An extra serving of beans prepared without fat will help reduce the risk of all the illnesses I've discussed.
- Sensible supplementation, outlined in the next section, will help.

A few habits can make the Longevity Diet even more effective. You've heard them before, but they're worth repeating.

- Eat fruit for dessert; for example, a slice of melon, half a mango, or a slice of watermelon. Fruit is cheaper in the long run than traditional desserts and provides all the protector substances.
- Snack on vegetables, fruits, and nuts. They provide protector substances.
- Always use whole-grain breads or rolls.
- Drink an 8-ounce glass of water first thing in the morning, thirty minutes before each meal, and once before bedtime.

If you follow the Smoker's Longevity Diet you'll get plenty of fiber, carotenoids, bioflavonoids, folic acid, and other nutrients that protect your health. However, you need more fiber and higher levels of many nutrients, such as vitamins E, C, and B complex, and the carotenoids. Therefore, it's fair for you to ask a question: Do I need supplements?

RDA VERSUS PROTECTOR NEED

Our bodies need vitamins C and E as protectors at higher levels than their RDA requirement. This higher level is needed because, as protectors, vitamins C and E don't serve as vitamins. They actually neutralize toxins, and each one is destroyed in the process. That's why the "protector function" is not always the same as the "vitamin function." For the same reason, we also need more protective beta carotene than is required to make vitamin A. There's no RDA for tocopherols other than alpha tocopherol, for carotenoids such as lycopene, or for other nutrients, such as fiber, so the protector function should be the criterion of need. At first it may seem as if the concepts here are at odds with the RDAs. They're not.

If you exceed the RDA by taking, say, up to over ten times the amount specified, you'll be free of toxicity symptoms *with two exceptions.* The two exceptions are vitamins A and D. Don't confuse beta carotene or other carotenoids with vitamin A. Beta carotene is converted to vitamin A in the body only as required. You can't get toxic levels of vitamin D from sunshine because your body has the built-in safety of its skin pigments. If you use vitamin D–fortified dairy products or calcium supplements, you'll be safe. There's a natural safety and regulated safety associated with vitamins A and D. Regulations that will limit the amount of vitamins A and D in supplements are pending. Serious abuse of vitamin A and vitamin D supplements, usually coupled with ignorance, creates a toxic situation. Use common sense.

When the RDAs were determined, protector functions were not taken into account. These protector functions have emerged because we live much longer, on average, than when scientists first started to assign nutritional need. In those days we didn't think of diseases such as cancer, cataracts, and emphysema as dietary issues. And no one thought about neutralizing toxins, such as nitrates, or excess ultraviolet light. Our longevity represents the triumphs of modern medicine. However, the protector function of nutrients and food components opens new horizons for nutritional biochemistry and personal responsibility.

DO YOU NEED SUPPLEMENTS?

As the twentieth century winds down, sensible supplements can help everyone, especially smokers. Compare supplements to pocket calculators. It's good to be able to calculate square roots by longhand, but using a calculator is more efficient use of your time. Supplements are a little like that. They don't substitute for the Smoker's Longevity Diet. They make it better. Diet will always be the foundation of health, and supplements make it just a little stronger. A survey of registered dieticians by the American Dietetic Association revealed that about 55 percent of them use food supplements. That's 10 percent more than the 45 percent of average folks who use them. Dieticians are the same people who say you can get what you need from a balanced diet. Although it sounds a little like the doctor who says to stop smoking while he lights up a cigarette, it isn't. It proves that the experts want to ensure the balanced diet they try to follow, or that they realize that stresses in our complex world impose greater nutrient demands on our bodies than food alone provides. They're also more aware of the protective power some nutrients provide, and they simply want to "hedge their bets." Supplements are an insurance policy for them and should be the same for you. Table 17.1 provides a list of basic, general supplements that will ensure that your basic nutrition won't be lacking.

Assess your own diet against the Smoker's Longevity Diet and what you've read here to see if you need more supplements. Calcium and magnesium are too bulky to satisfy the RDA in a supplement. Therefore, a separate calcium-magnesium supplement should be used along with the multivitamin-multimineral supplement.

SUPPLEMENTS BEYOND THE BASICS

I believe smokers, folks who live with smokers, and tobacco users need vitamins and nutrients above and beyond what the Smoker's Longevity Diet and a basic supplement provide. Consider the following.

TABLE 17.1
MULTIVITAMIN-MULTIMINERAL SUPPLEMENTS

Supplement	Company	Comments Per Tablet
Centrum	Lederle	100% U.S. RDA Calcium 16% Magnesium 25%
Dr. James Scala Signature Line	Nature's Sunshine Products	50% U.S. RDA Calcium 25% Magnesium 25%
Geritol Complete	Beechum Products	100% U.S. RDA Calcium 16% Magnesium 25%
Myadec	Parke Davis	100% U.S. RDA Calcium 7% Magnesium 25%
Theragran M	E.R. Squib and Sons	100% U.S. RDA Calcium 4% Magnesium 25%
Vita-Lea*	Shaklee Corporation	50% U.S. RDA Calcium 30% Magnesium 25%

*Available through independent distributors.

Vitamin C

If you take an additional 500 to 2,000 milligrams daily, you will have a sufficient excess of vitamin C to cover all the concepts I have introduced. Be sure the vitamin C supplement you buy contains bioflavonoids.

Vitamin E

Much research supports about 100 international units (IU) of vitamin E daily for average folks and about 400 IU for smokers. So, I think it's logical to start there with vitamin E supplements.

Beta Carotene

I would like to see a "carotene" supplement that contains a mixture of carotenoids, such as lycopene, and others. Until then, however, I urge you to take 25 milligrams of beta carotene daily. In addition to that, snack on carrots, tomatoes, and other red and yellow fruit.

Calcium

You should make sure you get 1,000 milligrams of calcium daily and up to 2,000 milligrams if you're past menopause. You can do it with milk and dairy products or calcium-magnesium supplements. (See Chapter 9.) These days there's no excuse for falling short in calcium.

B Complex

The most basic reason for a smoker to take extra B-complex vitamins is elevated metabolic rate, but there are other reasons; for instance, if you're under a lot of emotional or physical stress, or take medication (birth control pills, aspirin, high blood pressure medication, etc.). You can take as much as four to five times the RDA of these nutrients—400 or 500 percent of the RDA on the label. Select a complete B-complex supplement that is balanced with the RDAs of all the B vitamins. Don't be confused by the milligrams listed on the label, as they are different for each vitamin. Select your supplement according to the RDA, because that's what counts.

Fish Oil (EPA) or Flaxseed Oil

Even if you follow the Smoker's Longevity Diet, you can still benefit by taking extra fish oil—up to about 1,000 milligrams daily. Alternatively, or concurrently, put a tablespoon of flaxseed oil on your cereal each day or on your salad with the dressing. Flaxseed oil is tasteless, odorless, convenient, and inexpensive.

Garlic and Cruciferous Vegetables

Garlic supplements have been available for decades. I'm not certain that they are as effective as eating fresh garlic. Select "aged," not "chemically deodorized," garlic if you do choose a garlic supplement.

Cruciferous vegetable supplements are just appearing as I write this book. These supplements, made by freeze-drying cruciferous vegetables, should be effective. The freeze-drying process does not destroy important protector substances.

However, you still should eat both fresh garlic and cruciferous vegetables. Take the supplements for insurance.

A Waste of Money?

Whenever I'm asked if supplements are a waste of money, my reply is, "Compared to what?" I need a yardstick. Is it a waste compared to other things we spend money on? Consider the following examples. Every day Americans spend about the listed amount on these products.

- **Beer**: About 38¢ (34 gallons annually per capita).
- **Chocolates**: We eat 0.8 ounces per capita daily; that's 16¢ worth.
- **Cigarettes**: Every minute 1,631,000 cigarettes are lit. That's $1.18 daily per capita, and as a smoker, it's a lot more. In 1990, over 1,000,000 cigarettes were lit up every minute. At 12¢ each, that's over 69¢ a day per capita. Alternatively, it's $3.60 daily for the average 1.5 pack a day smoker.
- **Coffee**: The average adult drinks three cups each day, or about 45¢ worth.
- **Hair care**: The average woman spends over $1.00 daily.
- **Hot dogs**: They're loaded with nitrates and fat, and both help cancer along. We each eat 80 per year, at about 8¢ daily.
- **Soft drinks**: About 60¢ (7.8 ounces of soft drinks daily per capita).

I'm not telling you to quit using soft drinks, beer, coffee, or cigarettes. I like people's hair to look nice, and I like chocolate. However, don't tell me that something you can do that's positive for your health is a waste of money. It's actually cheaper to use vitamin C supplements than eat oranges.

MISCONCEPTIONS ABOUT SUPPLEMENTS

When I speak to folks in the United States and abroad about nutrition, I'm amazed by two very different groups of people who have misconceptions about nutrition for the same reasons. One group takes large amounts (megadoses) of food supplements. It's not uncommon for someone to tell me he takes 5 grams of vitamin C daily, or as many as ten to twenty different supplements. The other group has usually tried supplements but couldn't see a difference in how they felt, so they stopped. Neither group is particularly careful, or expert, about its diet.

Megavitamin users often think that vitamin supplements can make up for not eating a good diet. They try to separate food from nutrition. In short, they get pleasure from food and seek nutrition from pills. Many of these people think they can eat anything as long as they take copious quantities of supplements.

In contrast to the loyal megavitamin users, other people think that if they take some supplements today, tomorrow they'll be able to leap buildings in a single bound like Superman. These people expect to get the same quick results that a strong drug, prescribed for an illness, delivers. They often have a poor attitude about diet. Because they don't notice the effects of diet or supplements quickly, they usually don't bother taking either seriously. They lose out two ways.

ARE MEGADOSES THE ANSWER?

Nutrition is far from being an exact science. For instance, certain factors in food, such as the flavonoids, and in cruciferous vegetables seem to make vitamin C more effective or can replace it altogether. Similarly, there are about 350 other carotenoids in foods beside beta carotene. The roles of these factors are not well understood, but they're probably important. Therefore, taking extra vitamin C in pill form will certainly do some good, but eating an extra orange or kiwi fruit might prove even more beneficial.

NUTRITION IS A SLOW-MOTION TONIC

Unless you have a serious, diet-related health problem, you won't detect a significant physical change overnight from the Smoker's Longevity Diet, even if you use additional supplements. Improving your nutrition always pays, but the most powerful dividends, such as a longer life, accumulate slowly without notice. Nutrition is about wellness, not illness.

An aggressive program of self-health renewal includes diet, life-style changes, and sensible food supplements. People who want to see how well this entire plan works should keep a personal health diary for a month or two, in which they record daily how they feel, look, sleep, and wake up, and their energy level, regularity, and disposition. If you keep a diary like this you won't be disappointed, because you'll see results. A health diary is a good way to get in touch with your body and understand your feelings—you'll discover the best "you."

For example, people who follow a diet plan to lower blood pressure usually detect significant results in a week or ten days. And in four to eight weeks, many can stop using medication. In contrast, when people follow a dietary program to help arthritis, they usually get some results in ten days, mild results in about three or four weeks, but it requires six months for obvious improvements in mobility, inflammation, and pain. Even then, a person with arthritis seldom can stop taking some form of medication, at least occasionally. Similarly, smokers who follow the Smoker's Longevity Diet and add supplements will identify subtle but definite results within a few days, even though it's a lifetime commitment. For example, in a week or two fingernails usually become a little stronger with a healthy, pink color beneath the nail bed. This reflects better metabolism and circulation. People also notice, within a few days, that they sleep more soundly and wake up with more energy. In about a week, stamina improves and they feel more relaxed while having as much energy at the end of the day as at the beginning.

These changes are indications of better general health. They are subtle and accumulate so slowly that most people are unaware of them. What's worse, if you stop your nutrition commitment, the benefits will decline as slowly as they started, so even when they go away, they aren't noticed. You'll think it's normal.

Bowel regularity is the change that everyone experiences quickly. Within a few days of starting this plan, people start to notice a change in their bowel movements—they'll have one every twenty-four to thirty-six hours. As one couple said: "We stopped the daily laxative we used." In addition to feeling better, regularity also helps your complexion. The old saying, "an apple a day keeps the doctor away" began over 800 years ago, probably as a reflection of the good complexion that regularity produces.

Your health evolved to its present state over many years and is the sum total of heredity, environment, diet, life-style, and emotions, including all your good and bad habits. Therefore, the fact that you can notice an effect from diet within a few weeks or a month is truly spectacular. It shows how your body responds to a little nutritional support.

PUT THEORY INTO PRACTICE

Whenever I lecture on this diet, especially to medical students, I'm asked whether I myself follow it. Yes, I do. Then I'm asked how I proceed. In the next chapter I present some menus that put this plan into daily reality. I've even included an approximate calorie breakdown to prove you'll be eating better.

One characteristic I've noticed in successful executives is an ability to set priorities. And when it comes to our personal life, we're the top executive. The buck stops with the face you see in the mirror! What priority in our life can be put above our health? I don't know of a single one.

Let this diet become your eating habit and pass its concepts on to your loved ones. They will be rewarded with a longer and fuller life. You will be putting an important axiom into practice: *"Nutrition is preventive medicine and food is the vehicle of its practice."*

CHAPTER EIGHTEEN

SAMPLE MENUS FOR THE SMOKER'S LONGEVITY DIET

A fter I finished a lecture on dieting, a woman asked me, "When do I start?" "Immediately," I answered. This first instant of the rest of your life is the best time to start developing habits that will help you live longer and live better. And if you're like me, you'd like a few examples to get started. This show-me chapter will help you begin this worthwhile challenge.

MENUS: A GUIDELINE

I've used the Smoker's Longevity Diet and each chapter in this book to develop seven daily food plans that illustrate the versatility of the diet program. My objective is to stimulate your own creativity. Make a contest out of designing more imaginative and varied menus than mine, and be on your way to a longer, healthier life. It's a contest where everyone is a winner.

Note: In the sample menus, the numbers in parentheses indicate the calorie count for specific foods.

Serving sizes:

Dieticians, nutritionists, and food technologists use standard serving sizes. These sizes are expressed when necessary but are consistent with all recognized handbooks, especially *Bowes and Church's*, which is the most widely used. Some examples follow:

> Beverages (milk, juice, etc.): 6 ounces juice, 8 ounces milk

Yogurt: 8 ounces
Cereal: ½ cup serving
Fruit: a medium piece, such as an apple, or a banana
Vegetables: ½ cup cooked
Bread and rolls: 1 slice or 1 roll

If sugar is added to coffee, tea, etc.: 1 teaspoon = 15 calories. (I recommend not adding sugar or artificial sweeteners, but if a sweetener is used, I recommend natural sugar.)

SAMPLE MENUS FOR A WEEK

Day 1

Meal	Calories
Breakfast	
Glass of water	0
½ grapefruit	39
All Bran cereal (50) with low-fat milk (104), ½ sliced banana (52)	206
One slice whole-grain bread (61), toasted and buttered (36)	97
Tea or coffee, optional	0
Midmorning Snack	
Glass of water; coffee or tea	0
Peach yogurt	260
Carrots sticks	31
Lunch	
Glass of water	0
Bean soup	157
1 Whole-wheat roll (72) with butter (36)	108
Lettuce salad (4) with tomatoes (12), cucumber (4), green pepper (5), and onions (4), Italian dressing (14)	43
Steamed broccoli	12
Lime sherbet	135
Tea or coffee (optional)	0
Afternoon Snack	
Glass of water	0
Apple (81) with cheddar cheese (114)	195

Dinner

Glass of water	0
Broiled salmon with herbs	100
Baked potato (88) with sour cream and chives (26)	114
Steamed broccoflower	12
Salad (see lunch)	43
Low-fat ice cream (140) with sliced strawberries (22)	162
Tea or coffee, optional	0

Evening Snack

Pear	98

Day 1 Total	**1,812**

DAY 2

Breakfast

Glass of water	0
8 ounces orange juice (fresh squeezed)	111
Slice of cantaloupe	57
Oatmeal (109) with raisins (56), low-fat milk (104)	169
Whole-wheat English muffin (170), butter (36)	206
Tea or coffee, optional	0

Midmorning Snack

Glass of water	0
Bran muffin	112

Lunch

Glass of water	0
Tuna fish salad (172) sandwich on whole-wheat bread (140)	212
Carrot sticks	31
Coleslaw	42
Tea or coffee (optional)	0

Afternoon Snack

Glass of water	0
Pear (98) with feta cheese (75)	173

Dinner

Glass of water	0

Cheese ravioli with tomato sauce with onions, garlic, spices	284
Mixed salad greens (5) with tomatoes (12), green pepper (5), garbanzo beans (32), Italian dressing (14)	68
Dish of spinach	6
Cannoli	171
Tea or coffee, optional	0
Evening Snack	
Apple	81
Total Day 2	**1,723**

Day 3

Breakfast	
Glass of water	0
Orange-grapefruit juice	80
Sliced oranges and strawberries	55
Whole-wheat waffles (206) with maple syrup (50)	256
Tea or coffee, optional	0
Midmorning Snack	
Glass of water	0
Cheddar cheese (114) and grapes (75)	189
Lunch	
Glass of water	0
Salmon quiche	215
Triple-bean salad	90
Pear	98
Tea or coffee (optional)	0
Afternoon Snack	
Glass of water	0
Carrot and celery sticks	35
Dinner	
Glass of water	0
Stir-fried chicken with broccoli, broccoflower, red peppers, onion, garlic, ginger, and mushrooms	266
Rice	112

Mixed green salad (5) with water chestnuts (15), green onions (7), and mandarin oranges (23), Thousand Island dressing (24)	74
Apple-tapioca pudding	101
Tea or coffee, optional	0
Evening Snack	
Banana	105
Total Day 3	**1,676**

Day 4

Breakfast	
Glass of water	0
Slice of melon (57) with blueberries (41)	98
2 poached eggs (158) on whole-wheat toast (63)	221
1 slice lean ham	50
Tea or coffee, optional	0
Midmorning Snack	
Glass of water	0
Blueberry muffin	176
Lunch	
Glass of water	0
Curried chicken salad on lettuce	136
Banana bread	85
Frozen banana yogurt	143
Tea or coffee (optional)	0
Afternoon Snack	
Glass of water	0
Grapes	58
Dinner	
Glass of water	0
Halibut steak, broiled	119
Mixed green salad (5) with tomatoes (12), onions (7), red pepper (6), zesty tomato dressing (11)	38
Carrots	31
Asparagus	12

Rice	112
Apple strudel	96
Tea or coffee, optional	0
Evening Snack	
Brick cheese (105) and whole-wheat crackers (70)	175
Pear	98

Total Day 4	**1,648**

Day 5

Breakfast	
Glass of water	0
Sliced oranges, bananas, and kiwi fruit	72
Fiber One cereal (60) with low-fat milk (104)	164
Bran muffin (112), butter (36)	148
Tea or coffee, optional	0
Midmorning Snack	
Glass of water	0
Fruit yogurt	260
Lunch	
Glass of water	0
Lentil soup	69
Melted cheese and crab on English muffin	238
Mixed salad greens (5) with tomato (12) and cucumbers (4), zesty tomato dressing (11)	32
Brussels sprouts	30
Pear	98
Tea or coffee (optional)	0
Afternoon Snack	
Glass of water	0
Celery sticks (12) with peanut butter (47)	59
Carrot sticks	31
Dinner	
Glass of water	0
Zucchini lasagne with tomato sauce with onions, garlic, and herbs	189
Corn	89
Lemon, cabbage, carrot mold with lettuce	57

Crusty French bread, butter	81
Cheesecake	150
Tea or coffee, optional	0
Evening Snack	
Plum	36

Total Day 5	**1,803**

Day 6

Breakfast	
Glass of water	0
8 ounces orange juice (fresh squeezed)	111
½ papaya	59
Fiber One cereal (60) with low-fat milk (104) and blueberries (41)	205
Tea or coffee, optional	0
Midmorning Snack	
Glass of water	0
Fruit yogurt	260
Lunch	
Glass of water	0
Spinach salad with mushrooms, chopped egg, onion, bacon bits; oil, vinegar, and mustard dressing	218
Broiled salsify	46
Popover	90
Sliced peaches	66
Tea or coffee (optional)	0
Afternoon Snack	
Glass of water	0
Rice cakes (35) with cream cheese (98)	133
Dinner	
Glass of water	0
Filet of sole	80
Basil bean salad with onions, garlic	90
Rice pilaf	121
Spinach	6
Pumpkin pie	212
Tea or coffee, optional	0

Evening Snack

Pear	98
Dried apricots	83

Total Day 6	**1,878**

Day 7

Breakfast

Glass of water	0
Sliced peaches (37) with low-fat cottage cheese (41)	78
Whole-wheat pancakes (142) with blueberries (41) and maple syrup (50)	233
Tea or coffee, optional	0
Midmorning Snack	
Glass of water	0
Fruit yogurt	260
Dried apricots	83
Lunch	
Glass of water	0
Creamy carrot soup	149
Salmon salad with lettuce and tomato in pita bread	136
Raspberries	61
Tea or coffee (optional)	0
Afternoon Snack	
Glass of water	0
Applesauce wheat bar	134
Dinner	
Glass of water	0
Marinated lamb roast with garlic	180
Tossed greens (5) with sliced canned pears (50)	55
Small roasted potatoes	65
Green beans	22
Broccoli	23
Whole-wheat roll with butter	70
Lemon dream parfaits	176
Tea or coffee, optional	0

Evening Snack

Orange	65
Total Day 7	**1,790**

CALORIES COUNT

As you look over the menu plan, you'll notice that each food item has its approximate calorie count and the daily calories are totaled to prove that you won't get fat eating this way. In fact, I'll make a promise: If you're overweight now, and you start living by the Smoker's Longevity Diet, your weight will slowly drop to normal.

However, this isn't a weight-loss plan. It's a healthful, sensible way of eating. Any weight loss comes because you're eating a more bulky diet with less fat and less sugar. You'll feel full and won't get cravings.

HOW MANY CALORIES DO I NEED?

Placing calories alongside menus is good news for those who watch calories. It's bad news for those who don't, because natural curiosity raises a question: How many calories do I need each day?

Table 18.1 gives you an idea of how many calories you need, depending on how you spend your day. Most people lead lives somewhere between sedentary and moderately active, and a smoker burns more calories than average nonsmokers. I've put these two extremes of calorie use together for you in the table so you can estimate your own needs.

Just keep a few things in mind. We're all different and we all use different amounts of energy for the same processes. In addition, we each digest and absorb our food a little differently. So, if two people follow this diet plan, one might lose a little weight and the other will stay the same. It's highly unlikely that you would gain weight on this plan because it calls for a lot of bulk (fruit and vegetables) and is low in fat.

TABLE 18.1
DAILY CALORIE* BALANCE FOR AVERAGE PEOPLE WHO SMOKE

		Age 30 Activity Level		Age 50 Activity Level	

Women

Height	Weight	Sedentary	Moderately Active	Sedentary	Moderately Active
5'2"	130	1,840	2,150	1,745	2,026
5'5"	145	2,005	2,335	1,895	2,210
5'7"	155	2,120	2,475	2,005	2,335

Men

Height	Weight	Sedentary	Moderately Active	Sedentary	Moderately Active
5'10"	180	2,505	2,919	2,385	2,780
6'0"	190	2,604	3,035	2,480	2,900
6'2"	200	2,730	3,180	2,605	3,030

*Calories are always approximate and were calculated as follows:
A. Basal metabolic rates (BMR) from body surface-area measurements
B.   Activity level
    Sedentary person: 0.2 times BMR
    Moderately active person: 0.4 times BMR
C. Calories lost to assimilation   0.1 times BMR + activity
D. Calories expended due to effect of nicotine on BMR   0.05 times BMR
    Total daily calories = A + B + C + D
    Sedentary (mostly sitting): e.g., secretary, computer clerk
    Moderately active: e.g., nurse, waiter or waitress, driver
    Most people fall between these two extremes. However, a carpenter (active) would be about 0.5 times BMR.

Exercise: If you exercise as recommended in this book, you will burn an additional 200 to 400 calories daily depending on your size, vigor of exercise, and time spent.

The weights given will undoubtedly differ from those you find on "ideal" weight and height charts supplied by insurance companies, which will be about 7 percent less in weight. All ideal weights are guidelines, so I selected these as average and not necessarily ideal weights. If you maintain a weight within the "ideal" given by an insurance company, that is excellent.

SERVING SIZE

In writing menu plans and preparing meals, I've used standard portions, such as ½ cup or 3.5 ounces, or practical portions, like one apple. This allows you to use standard food composition handbooks, recipe books, or nutritional labels on packaged foods to make your own meal plans. You can adjust serving size and substitute foods if gaining or losing weight is an objective. Just reducing your serving size makes it the best weight-loss plan you'll ever follow.

Suppose a six-foot four-inch, 200-pound linebacker is married to a five-foot four-inch fashion model who weighs 120 pounds. If they both eat the same meals according to this plan, serving size will keep him from shrinking and her from becoming huge. His servings will naturally be larger than hers. He might have two pears to her half pear, or perhaps take a double serving of fish. The size of the portions doesn't matter, because the food composition is the same.

SUPPLEMENTS

If you're like most people you're still wondering: My doctor said I can get everything from a balanced diet. Besides, he said they are a waste of money.

My intention is for you to make your own decision on supplements. If you decide for yourself, you'll be firm in your decision and won't need to be concerned with critics that advocate one side or the other.

BALANCED DIET

Most Americans and all smokers don't eat a balanced diet. I hope that from now on more of us will. When I teach nutrition to medical students, I hand them a copy of a balanced diet similar to the one in Chapter 17. One student is always sure to ask: "Who eats like that?" I tell them about 10 percent of the population based on the data in Table 18.2.

Less than 10 percent of nonsmokers eat a balanced diet. No one knows precisely what a balanced diet would be for smokers. The Smoker's Longevity Diet is an excellent, basic start, but it's never going to have enough of vitamins C and

TABLE 18.2
AMERICA'S FOOD HABITS

Food	Approximate Percentage of Americans
No fruit	20
No vegetables	27
No fruit or vegetables	7
No salad	20
Salad less than once weekly	60

Daily Consumption	Ounces
Beef per capita daily	3.5
Chicken per capita daily	3.2
Fish per capita daily	0.2

E. If you don't eat lots of carrots or pumpkin, it won't have nearly enough beta carotene, and even nonsmokers can't get the level of omega-3 oils they should really have. All these shortfalls can be made up by using supplements, but the supplements won't make up for the food. The bottom line is: you need both.

In the June 1992 issue of the *Journal of the American Dietetic Association*, a thorough dietary analysis of 1,120 women aged nineteen through fifty was published. This analysis was conducted six times over one year and included women who ate at home, away from home, and some who combined both. All of these women fell significantly below the RDA for all nutrients followed in the study, including fiber, calcium, copper, zinc, vitamin A, and folic acid. They achieved the RDA for vitamin C. Their K factor was less than 1.

This confirms that average people don't eat a balanced diet and that sensible supplementation can make up for many dietary shortfalls. Only good food selection and preparation can correct the K factor.

Epilogue

Nicotine Patches and Nicotine Gum

Nicotine patches and nicotine gum help people overcome the addictive nature of nicotine, or to quit smoking; it works by slowly "weaning" the addicted person from high levels of nicotine. For example, it takes smokers from the level in three packs of cigarettes daily to a level so low so that they won't notice the absence of nicotine in their bloodstream.

Nicotine patches and gum help you quit best in conjunction with a behavioral modification program conducted by an expert counselor. This need for counseling is proof that nicotine addiction has either changed you, or has filled a void that, now emptied, you must learn to live with again. This is indirect proof that the effects of nicotine benefit some people, and they are usually those who become addicted when they start smoking or chewing tobacco.

Some people try smoking but never develop the habit. I'm one of those people. I tried smoking while in the military service, but it didn't do anything for me. Consequently, what was pleasurable for many of my friends was not for me. My experience shows that we are as different on the inside as we are on the outside.

Outward differences are obvious: size, shape, color, and all the characteristics that make each of us unique. If you could look at a person's kidneys, heart, and other organs, you'd see distinct differences, just like the external variations. Our brain is also unique because personality, which is 70 percent heredity, results from the arrangement of brain cells and the biochemicals they produce and how they pass from one to another. In short, we're different right down to each of the 13 trillion cells in our body.

Just as each person is dependent for survival on vitamins from plants, it's not surprising that some of us can get along better if we get other materials from plants, such as nicotine and caffeine. If they have a psychological effect on us, we often, but not always, call these other substances "drugs." For example, most governments have declared cocaine a drug, but not caffeine.

Let's put smoking aside for a moment and look at the drug nicotine. Nicotine ranks in addictive capacity with drugs such as caffeine, alcohol, cocaine, heroin, and many others. How would we use nicotine if we had never learned to smoke or chew tobacco? Would there be an illegal nicotine cartel? Would there be an illegal trade in nicotine? What about caffeine, if there was no such thing as coffee or tea?

Even though nicotine patches and gum have been designed to help people stop smoking, it's reasonable to assume that some people may choose nicotine as a life-style option along with the many who use caffeine and alcohol. Should we allow people to use nicotine patches in place of smoking or chewing tobacco?

CHEWING TOBACCO

As the decline in smoking continues, more chewing tobacco is used. Recently, a 7-Eleven store owner said it simply: "I can't keep chewing tobacco on the shelf." Chewing tobacco provides a satisfying nicotine fix similar to smoking. Its use creates another argument for giving nicotine a benign drug status so that it might be safely obtained in gum or patches. We could avoid some of the diseases tobacco causes, while recognizing that nicotine makes some people feel better from day to day. And these tobacco sources do not produce second-hand smoke.

Although chewing tobacco has not been studied nearly as extensively as smoking, there is substantial evidence showing that some of its effects are worse than smoking. Therefore, the advice in this book for smokers applies even more for tobacco chewers. Indeed, I would urge tobacco chewers to double up on many of the health suggestions I gave for smokers, and that's still no substitute for quitting.

ADDITIONAL READINGS AND SOURCES

This reading list emphasizes review articles, symposium publications, and a few papers that are especially pertinent to the points and plans discussed in this book. Serious students will glean important information from the works cited.

FOOD COMPOSITION

Bowes and Church's Food Values of Portions Commonly Used, 15th ed. revised by Jean A. T. Pennington (Philadelphia: Lippincot, 1989).

GENERAL NUTRITION

Whitney, E., E. Hamilton, and A. Rolfes. *Understanding Nutrition* (St. Paul: West, 1990).

CHAPTER I

Chu, S. Y., et. al. "Cigarette Smoking and the Risk of Breast Cancer." *American Journal of Epidemiology* 131, no. 2 (1990): 244–253.

Farrow, D. C., and S. Davis. "Risk of Pancreatic Cancer in Relation to Medical History and the Use of Tobacco, Alcohol, and Coffee." *International Journal of Cancer* 45, no. 5 (1990): 816–820.

Glantz, S. A., and W. W. Parmley. "Passive Smoking and Heart Disease: Epidemiology, Physiology, and Biochemistry." *Circulation* 83, no. 1 (1991): 1–12.

Morabia, A., and E. L. Wynder. "Dietary Habits of Smokers, People Who Never Smoked, and Ex-smokers." *American Journal of Clinical Nutrition* 52, no. 5 (1990): 933–937.

La Vecchia, C., and E. Negri. "The Role of Alcohol in Oesophageal Cancer in Non-smokers, and of Tobacco in Non-drinkers." *International Journal of Cancer* 43, no. 5 (1989): 784–785.

Oliver, M. F. "Cigarette Smoking, Polyunsaturated Fats, Linoleic Acid, and Coronary Heart Disease." *Lancet* 1, no. 8649 (1989): 1241–1243.

Persson, P. G., A. Ahlbom, and G. Hellers. "Inflammatory Bowel Disease and Tobacco Smoke—A Case-Control Study." *Gut* 31, no. 12 (1990): 1377–1381.

"Proceedings of the Third International Conference on the Prevention of Human Cancer." *Preventive Medicine* 18, no. 5 (September 1989): 553–739.

Recommended Dietary Allowances, 10th ed. (Washington, D.C.: Food and Nutrition Board of the National Academy of Sciences, 1989).

Spiller, Gene A., and James Scala, eds. *New Protective Roles for Selected Nutrients* (New York: Alan R. Liss, 1989).

Stemmermann, G. N., et al. "Impact of Diet and Smoking on Risk of Developing Intestinal Mataplasia of the Stomach." *Digestive Diseases and Sciences* 35, no. 4 (1990): 433–438.

Subar, A. F., L. C. Harlan, and M. E. Mattson. "Food and Nutrient Intake Differences Between Smokers and Non-smokers in the U.S." *American Journal of Public Health* 80, no. 11 (1990): 1323–1329.

Sumiyoshi, H., and M. J. Wargovich. "Garlic (Allium Sativum): A Review of Its Relationship to Cancer." *Asia Pacific Journal of Pharmacology* 4 (1989): 133–140.

CHAPTER 2

Brown, L. M., et al., "Environmental Factors and High Risk of Esophageal Cancer Among Men in Coastal South Carolina." *Journal of the National Cancer Institute* 80, no. 20 (1988): 1620–1625.

Byers, T. E., et al., "Diet and Lung Cancer Risk, Findings from the Western New York Diet Study." *American Journal of Epidemiology* 125, no. 3 (1987): 351–363.

Dormandy, T. L. "Free-Radical Pathology and Medicine." *Journal of the Royal College of Physicians of London* 23, no. 4 (October 1989): 221–227.

Garn, S. M., and W. R. Leonard. "What Did Our Ancestors Eat?" *Nutrition Reviews* 47, no. 11 (November 1989): 337–345.

Halliwell, B. "Tell Me About Free Radicals, Doctor." *Journal of the Royal Society of Medicine* 82, no. 12 (December 1989): 747–752.

"Proceedings of the Third International Conference on the Prevention of Human Cancer." *Preventive Medicine* 18, no. 5 (September 1989): 553–739.

Schectman, G., J. C. Byrd, and R. Hoffmann. "Ascorbic Acid Requirements for Smokers: Analysis of a Population Survey." *American Journal of Clinical Nutrition* 53 (1991): 1466–1470.

CHAPTER 3

Aoki, K., et al. "Smoking, Alcohol Drinking and Serum Carotenoids Levels." *Japanese Journal of Cancer Research* 78, no. 10 (1987): 1049–1056.

Bendich, A., and L. J. Machlin. "Safety of Oral Intake of Vitamin E." *American Journal of Clinical Nutrition* 48 (1988): 612–619.

Bendich, A., and J. A. Olson. "Biological Actions of Carotenoids." *FASEB Journal* 3, no. 8 (June 1989): 1927–1932.

Chow, C. K., et al. "Lower Levels of Vitamin C and Carotenes in Plasma of Cigarette Smokers." *Journal of the American College of Nutrition* 5, no. 3 (1986): 305–312.

Fan, A. M., and K. W. Kizer. "Selenium, Nutritional, Toxicological and Clinical Aspects." *Western Journal of Medicine* 153, no. 2 (August 1990): 160–167.

Gey, K. F., G. B. Brubacher, and H. B. Stahelin. "Plasma Levels of Antioxidant Vitamins in Relation to Ischemic Heart Disease and Cancer." *American Journal of Clinical Nutrition* 45 (1987): 1368–1377.

Keith, R. E., and S. B. Mossholder. "Ascorbic Acid Status of Smoking and Nonsmoking Adolescent Females." *Interna-*

tional Journal of Vitamin and Nutrition Research 56, no. 4 (1986): 363–366.

Wald, N. J., et al. "Serum Beta-Carotene and Subsequent Risk of Cancer: Results from the BUPA Study." *British Journal of Cancer* 57, no. 4 (1988): 428–433.

Willett, W. C. "Vitamin A and Lung Cancer." *Nutrition Reviews* 48, no. 5 (May 1990): 201–211.

Ziegler, R. G. "A Review of Epidemiologic Evidence That Carotenoids Reduce the Risk of Cancer." *Journal of Nutrition* 119 (1989): 116–122.

CHAPTER 5

Rose, D. P. "Dietary Fiber and Breast Cancer." *Nutrition and Cancer* 13, no 5. 1 and 2 (1990): 1–8.

Spiller, G. A., ed. *CRC Handbook of Dietary Fiber in Human Nutrition* (Boca Raton, FL: CRC Press, 1986).

Stemmermann, G. N., et al. "Impact of Diet and Smoking on Risk of Developing Intestinal Mataplasia of the Stomach." *Digestive Diseases and Sciences* 35, no. 4 (1990):443–438.

Trock, B., E. Lanca, and J. Greenwald. "Dietary Fiber, Vegetables and Colon Cancer." *National Cancer Institute* 82, no. 8 (April 1990): 650–661.

Wu-Williams, A. H., M. C. Yu, and T. M. Mack. "Life-Style, Workplace, and Stomach Cancer by Subsite in Young Men of Los Angeles County." *Cancer Research* 50, no. 9 (1990): 2569–2576.

CHAPTER 6

Dyerberg, J. "The Eskimo Experience." *n-3 News* 1, no. 1 (January 1986): 1–4.

Garn, S. M., and W. R. Leonard. "What Did Our Ancestors Eat?" *Nutrition Reviews* 47, no. 11 (November 1989): 337–345.

Simopoulos, A. P., R. R. Kifer, and R. E. Martin, eds. *Health*

Effects of Polyunsaturated Fatty Acids in Seafoods. (New York: Academic Press, 1986).

Turini, M. E., K. B. Tapan, and M. T. Clandinin. "Prostaglandins-Diet-Cancer." *Nutrition Research* 10, no. 7 (July 1990): 819–827.

Wan, J. M-F., M. P. Haw, and G. L. Blackburn. "The Interaction Between Nutrition and Inflammation: An Overview." *Proceedings of the Nutrition Society* 48, no. 3 (September 1989): 315–335.

Whichelow, M. J., S. W. Erzinclioglu, and B. D. Cox. "A Comparison of the Diets of Non-smokers and Smokers." *British Journal of Addiction* 86, no. 1 (1991): 71–81.

Whichelow, M. J., J. F. Golding, and F. P. Treasure. "Comparison of Some Dietary Habits of Smokers and Non-smokers." *British Journal of Addiction* 83, no. 3 (1988): 295–304.

CHAPTER 7

Scala, James. *The High Blood Pressure Relief Diet* (New York: NAL, 1988).

CHAPTER 8

Gey, K. F., G. B. Brubacher, and H. B. Stahelin. "Plasma Levels of Antioxidant Vitamins in Relation to Ischemic Heart Disease and Cancer." *American Journal of Clinical Nutrition* 45 (1987): 1368–1377.

Kowalski, Robert A. *The 8-Week Cholesterol Cure* (New York: Harper & Row, 1990).

The Surgeon General's Report on Nutrition and Health (Washington, DC: U.S. Government Printing Office, 1988).

CHAPTER 9

Gallager, J. C. "The Pathogenesis of Osteoporosis." *Bone and Mineral* 9, no. 3 (June 1990): 215–227.

Matkovic, V. "Factors That Influence Peak Bone Mass Formation." *American Journal of Clinical Nutrition* 52, no. 5 (November 1990): 878–888.

CHAPTER 10

Bailey, L. B. "The Role of Folate in Human Nutrition." *Nutrition Today* 25, no. 5 (September/October 1990): 12–18.

Benowitz, N. L., S. M. Hall, and G. Modin. "Persistent Increase in Caffeine Concentrations in People Who Stop Smoking." *British Medical Journal* 298, no. 6680 (1989): 1075–1076.

Brooke, O. G., et al. "Effects on Birth Weight of Smoking, Alcohol, Caffeine, Socioeconomic Factors, and Psychosocial Stress." *British Medical Journal* 298, no. 6676 (1989): 795–801.

Khoury, J. F., M. Gomez-Farias, and J. Mulinare. "Does Maternal Cigarette Smoking During Pregnancy Cause Cleft Lip and Palate in Offspring?" *American Journal of Diseases of Children* 143, no. 3 (1989): 333–337.

Milunsky, A., et al. "Multivitamin/Folic Acid Supplement in Early Pregnancy Reduces the Prevalence of Neural Tube Defects." *Journal of the American Medical Association* 262, no. 20 (1989): 2847–2852.

Rose, J. E. "Cigarette Smoking Blocks Caffeine-Induced Arousal." *Alcohol and Drug Research* 7, no. 1 (1987): 49–55.

Rubin, D. H., et al. "Effect of Passive Smoking on Birth-Weight." *Lancet* 11, no. 18504 (1986): 415–417.

Shiono, P. H., M. A. Klebanoff, and G. G. Rhoads, "Maternal Smoking Affects Length of Gestation." *Journal of the American Medical Association* 255, no. 1 (1986): 82–84.

CHAPTER 12

Cooper, Kenneth H. *Running Without Fear.* (New York: Bantam Books, 1986).

Klesges, R. C., et al. "Smoking Status: Effects on the Dietary

Intake, Physical Activity, and Body Fat of Adult Men." *American Journal of Clinical Nutrition* 51, no. 1 (1990): 784–789.

Troisi, R. J., J. W. Heinold, P. S. Vokonas, and S. T. Weiss. "Cigarette Smoking, Dietary Intake, and Physical Activity: Effects on Body Fat Distribution—The Normative Aging Study." *American Journal of Clinical Nutrition* 53 (1991): 1104–1111.

Yanker, Gary D. *The Complete Book of Exercise Walking.* (Chicago: Contemporary Books, 1983).

CHAPTERS 13, 14, AND 15

Haberman, Fredric, and Denise Fortino. *Your Skin* (New York: Berkley Books, 1986).

Novick, Nelson Lee. *Saving Face* (Los Angeles: The Body Press, 1986).

CHAPTER 16

Auervach, O., and L. Garfinkel. "Histologic Changes in Pancreas in Relation to Smoking and Coffee-Drinking Habits." *Digestive Diseases and Sciences* 31, no. 10 (1986): 1014–1020.

Gordon, T., and J. T. Doyle. "Effects of Alcohol and Smoking on Weight, Blood Pressure, and Blood Lipids." *Archives of Internal Medicine* 146, no. 2 (1986): 262–265.

Robinson, S., and D. A. York. "The Effect of Cigarette Smoking on the Thermic Response to Feeding." *International Journal of Obesity* 10, no. 5 (1986): 407–417.

Rosengren, A., L. Wilhilmsen, and H. Wedel. "Separate and Combined Effects of Smoking and Alcohol Abuse in Middle-aged Men." *Acta Medica Scandinavica* 223, no. 2 (1988): 111–118.

Siegel, Ronald K. *Intoxication: Life in Pursuit of Artificial Paradise* (New York: E. P. Dutton, 1989).

Williamson, D. F., et al. "Smoking Cessation and Severity of

Weight Gain in a National Cohort." *New England Journal of Medicine* 324, no. 11 (1991): 739–745.

CHAPTER 17

Haines, P. S., et al., "Eating Patterns and Energy and Nutrient Intakes of U.S. Women." *Journal of the American Dietetic Association* 92 (1992): 698–704.